Peak In

How to fight CEBV, Candida,
Herpes Simplex Viruses
and other immuno-suppressed Conditions
and... Win!

Luc De Schepper M.D. PhD. C.A.

From the same author:

- "Acupuncture Within Everyone's Reach" (1981)
- "Acupuncture for the Practitioner" (1985)
- "Candida, the Symptoms, the Causes, the Cure" (1986)

Dedicated to Yolanda

Library of Congress Catalog Card Number 88-093079

ISBN 0-9614734-2-8

The information in this book is not intended as medical advice. Its intention is solely informational and educational. It is assumed that the reader will consult a medical or health professional should the need for one be warranted.

ACKNOWLEDGMENTS

A work like this is the result of love and teamwork between doctor and patients. Therefore, all my patients have contributed to this book. Some of them have stood out. This book would not be the same without the editing work of my good friends David Horowitz (writer of "The Kennedy's") and Rose Friend. Both have been extremely encouraging and their professional advise was invaluable. The drawings are the result of the talents of Shay Marlowe and my beloved Yolanda. My friend Richard Lefevre used all his talents to format the book and made it as good-looking as it is. The cover was done by the talented Venke Blyberg.

Anyone afflicted by these diseases should consult a nutritional, holistic oriented doctor. I want to thank my patients for confining in me, for working with me and showing their confidence and hope. Without them, this book would not be possible. I feel very fortunate to have my patients as my friends, for having me taught so much about suffering, compassion and love. Hopefully, this book will give hope to millions of sufferers and a return to a healthy, fulfilling life.

Dr. Luc De Schepper
2901 Wilshire Boulevard
Suite 435
Santa Monica, CA 90403
(213) 828-4480

TABLE OF CONTENTS

3

4

INTRODUCTION

The 20th Century has witnessed the greatest technicological strides: the conquering of space, the exploration of the deepest oceans, ingenious computers that gather data faster than our mind can comprehend. Gone are the days of dawn to dusk labor, of low wages and no vacations -- a dream come true. A cloudless sky. Almost. Just when mankind has begun to enjoy the free time created by scientific progress, a new enemy has appeared to haunt us: epidemic disease. I hear you say: "Did we not also make enormous progress in medicine? Have we not produced 'miracle drugs' to combat all kinds of infectious agents and to wipe out such scourges as diptheria, small pox and cholera? Are we not on the threshold of conquering the other diseases that have plagued mankind?" We did, we are -- or at least we thought so. For a long time we felt rather comfortable with our medical arsenal, making great strides in bio-chemistry, inventing one "magic bullet" after another.

But now, suddenly, there is AIDS -- a viral killer which has frustrated even the most advanced bio-engineering techniques in the efforts to develop a cure. And not only AIDS. It is only recently that we have begun to realize that there are other enemies similar to the AIDS virus attacking our immune systems on an epidemic scale. In the last decades alone we have seen millions of people suffering from an array of immune disorders: Herpes Simplex Viruses, Hepatitis A and B Virus and parasites. And autoimmune disorders, affecting smaller numbers of people but no less destructive in their effects: Multiple Sclerosis, Lupus Erythomatosis, rheumatoid Arthritis, Colitis Ulcerosa and Crohn's disease, just to name a few. In these diseases, the body turns against its own tissues.

All these conditions have been around for a long time, yet no cure has been found. Under the impact of AIDS we have begun to realize that our batting average with other immune diseases has not been impressive. We don't have a cure for Herpes Simplex, hepatitis, Epstein Barr Virus, to mention the most pandemic among them. We have no treatment for viral diseases period.

The medical profession, in general, takes the view that people who fall prey to these conditions pretty much will suffer from them for the rest of their lives. The price the patient pays in terms of a depressed immune system is one that can be lived with, in the absence of a cure. However, the suffering of such patients aside, in the presence of the AIDS pandemic which threatens the immune system with total collapse, even a 5% decrease in the strength of the body's securety system may be decisive. It is estimated that tens of millions of Americans now suffer from EBV and Herpes Simplex. It is a matter of concern that these viruses are raging out of control in the bodies of the general population preparing the way for more deadly intruders.

The symptoms of those who suffer from these diseases are simple yet frightening. Take Sue, for example. She was 27 years old, sportive, outgoing, with endless energy. One day, this energy was gone. Her symptoms puzzled the many doctors she consulted, yet not one came up with a plausible reason. Numerous medications were prescribed, most of them with negative, even aggravating results. Yet, the only event that seemed to trigger this condition, was a broad spectrum antibiotic which she took for 14 days, and which had been prescribed for a flu-like condition.

Then there is Paul, a professor of ophtalmology at a renowned Californian university. He worked together with two other colleagues in a private office. It turned out to be a very bad relationship, in which he felt his colleagues were betraying him. Two months later, he came down with chronic fatigue, experiencing a decrease in memory and concentration, muscle pains and severe food allergies. When he suggested correctly that he might be suffering from Epstein Barr Virus, the university stopped sending him patients. His colleagues thought he had lost his mind, and didn't want anything to do with him.

Jill was another case. A bright student, excelling in swimming, skiing and tennis, she enjoyed perfect health until she started working at a job she hated, to supply her with enough income to get her through school. Before two months went by she found herself overcome with incredible fatigue, unable to cope with any daily stress and no desire for any of her regular activities. It took her more than a year to regain some of her old skills and to deal with her demanding studies.

It is common for us to see young college students whose grades have dropped from "A's to C's without any "noticeable reason." All of a sudden, they can't concentrate anymore, a "brainfog" seems to become a second nature. Frustrated parents bring them from one doctor to another, yet no one seems to have an answer. "It must be those teenage years," "Maybe my children are on drugs," are frequently heard comments. These young victims feel powerless and ultimately without support from their loved ones.

I have seen thousands of such cases in my practice, all with similar stories, symptoms and histories of ever more frustrating previous treatments. I feel sympathy for the millions of victims, manufactured daily by our polluted environment and artificial food intake and by uninformed doctors, who cover themselves by dismissing these immuno-suppressed diseases as "fad" conditions. Finally, these sufferers are overcome with another deadly disease: despair. Their condition overwhelms them, leaving them open to total catastrophe.

It took the Western medical world 10 years to accept the diagnosis of chronic Epstein Barr virus, and even now, many doctors discount this diagnosis, leaving millions of people in despair. Why this attitude? Let's face it. Nobody wants to be confronted with a situation where no help can be offered. It is easier to say, "It's all in your head." It takes the pressure away from the doctor who can shift the responsibility back to the patient. Even when accepting the diagnosis, doctors feel helpless, ignorant and saddened by this mysterious illness. Oh yes! We give it other fancy names, like "Chronic Fatigue Syndrome," mainly to express the unknown pathological factors involved. But naming a disease is not a cure.

Epstein Barr Virus has finally gotten its share of attention in the media, yet an even more vicious and widespread condition, CANDIDA, has overwhelmed millions of people. It is estimated that 20 million women suffer from vaginal yeast infections. Yet this is only the tip of the iceberg. The vaginal yeast discharge is only one symptom of this illness. The real number of these victims is much higher and does not exclude by any means the male population! In my estimation, Candida Albicans, a vicious yeast cell, plays a key role in the pathogenesis of the so-called "Chronic Fatigue Syndrome." At least 75% of yeast sufferers will have at the same time a pathological level of Epstein Barr Virus. And it does not stop there. From experience, I can say that it is extremely difficult, if not impossible, to find a person between the ages of 20 and 45 who does not suffer from either Candida, CEBV, Herpes Simplex I or II (the sexual form). Most of the victims, in fact, have to fight several of these conditions simultaneously. Can you imagine the immense battle of your immune system with these tiny invaders? Can you anticipate the strain on your adrenals, your whole endocrine system? And can you visualize the eventual outcome: a total breakdown of the immune system.

There is an ominous message in these facts. We think of AIDS as our ultimate enemy. But the real enemy is already within us, striking millions, weakening millions of us and allowing more deadly viruses to invade us. It is the Trojan horse that has entered our walled city. We are desperately looking for superweapons against AIDS, while we lose the battle against its advanced guard and family surrogates. I am not optimistic about the final outcome of the siege because too many elements -- in our environment, in the way we live -- have to change for us to win, and most of the time we are still busy making things worse. It is frightening to see the victims of Candida and CEBV coming from younger and younger segments of the population. A girl was brought to my practice who was 18 months old. She was suffering from a vaginal yeast infection because she had already been on antibiotics for 14 months. This is simply criminal. The life of this child was crippled before it had started. This child will crave sugar, become hyperactive, be given Ritalin and then classified as a "hyperactive" child who exhibited impossible behavior from birth. And yet, it is we who are responsible.

What excesses have led to these fearful epidemics? Why are we losing ground to diseases that were non-existant before? What have we done to ourselves and our world to make this happen?

This book will explore at length the answers to these and other questions, including what can be done to deal with the problem and rescue us from the situation we ourselves have created. But here is a thumbnail sketch of what has happened -- the change in the conditions of our lives that has produced this crisis.

In the first place, we have changed what we eat. Take a quick look at the American diet. It is low in fiber, low in protein and high in sugars, simple carbohydrates and fat. If food and drinks do not taste sweet, we think it's weird and add chemicals like saccharin and nutrasweet. Yet, our ancestors had only natural sweets from berries. They did not know the pleasures of our fat-loaded dairy products -- ice cream, milk, cheese and butter -- and ate only the flesh of animals that make up the leanest meat of our supermarkets. The results of our modern diet are devastating: atherosclerotic heart disease and stroke, hypertension, colon cancer, obesity, dental cavities and many other degenerative diseases of civilization are rampant.

We are not only messing around with our food; we are also playing God with nature. The "Greenhouse effect" and the disappearance of the ozone layer are two acute problems created by our determination to pollute our environment. The greenhouse effect is a global warming caused by pollutants in the atmosphere. The ozone layer protects us against the ultra violet radiation of the sun. Pictures taken by satellites show a "black hole" in the ozone layer above the South pole, which has already increased the incidence of skin cancer.

Another major change in our environment is the introduction of the very miracle drugs that have aided us in the battle against disease. "Iatrogenic" or "Doctor-induced conditions", are high on the list of medical problems in every developed country. They have resulted in addictions, immuno-suppressed conditions and a whole array of new diseases.

Technology has also proved to be a two-edged sword. Just

when we thought that the high technology we created would bring us more free time, more joy and relaxation, the contrary is the case. Everybody seems to feel obliged to work more, children do not get enough attention and are put in boarding schools and day-care centers, career goals dominate the household picture more and more, and spouses cannot communicate with each other. Modern living has become high-stress living. Emotional traumas and daily stress are the triggering factor in the suppression of the immune system.

Each year in the United States, 600,000 people die from cancer, in spite of our longterm, billion dollar research. The research is focussed on the fabrication of new medications and drugs; very little effort is put into educating the public about prevention. And I don't mean the annual examinations for cancer which are helpful. I mean the necessary changes in life-style and diet, the only really practical therapy and defense.

It will take more than some new "magic bullets" to repair the damage we are doing to the complex systems in our bodies that protect us from disease. None of these immune-suppressed diseases will be corrected without taking lifestyle, dietary and environmental factors into account.

In the following pages, I have outlined a picture of how the body's immune system works, and explained how to protect it and keep it strong, so that it, in turn, can take good care of us and keep us healthy throughout a lifetime. The immuno-suppressed diseases EBV, CMV, Candida Albicans, AIDS and Parasites are discussed in detail. A natural therapeutic approach to all of them is explained in a manner, so that everybody, healthy or sick, can benefit from this book. May it be the beginning of a more conscientious and healthy life.

1

THE IMMUNE SYSTEM

1. HOW IT WORKS

Ten years ago, the words, "immune system" were rarely heard. Immunology was a stepchild of medecine, looked upon with little, if any interest. Yet, of all the marvels of the human body, perhaps the most mysterious and indispensable is the immune system. Without it there could be no human life for very long. This marvellous system functions independently to keep us alive and well. Treated with respect and care, it stands guard 24 hours a day over our health and our very survival. Today, although still not very well understood, the words, "immune system", are known to most everyone. The reason -- a now infamous virus called AIDS.

AIDS, a new enemy that virulently attacks our immune system. An enemy which has produced fear and even paranoia. Anyone losing weight becomes suspicious. The presence of lymph nodes in the neck area and recurrent infections is worrying. The more courageous ones ask for the blood test, HIV. If the test is negative, the feeling of relief is only temporary. The doctor is asked, "How can I protect myself?" The usual answer is to refrain from promiscuous sex and use condoms and spermicidal cream. This of course is good advice, but rather like putting the horse before the cart. The real question which both doctor and patient should address is, "How can I keep my immune system strong under the daily, relentless attacks by millions of unseen ennemies?"

One reason that all of a sudden we are paying more attention to the immune system is that immunology was a backwater of medicine until the discovery of powerful new laboratory methods; made it possible to probe the complexity of the system. A miracle of evolution, it is an example of a perfect democracy, in which each member performs its particular task without being controlled by a superior central organ. It is our immune system that provides a 24 hour security system, always on the alert for viruses, harmful bacteria, fungi, protozoa, pollens and even malignant cells. Every second of every day battles rage within our bodies. Most of the time, we don't have the slightest idea about the incessant wars against these warriors which are too tiny to see. Did you know that 200 million AIDS viruses would fit on the tip of a needle? Yet this virus is able to neutralize much larger cells.

At our disposition, we have legions of potent defenders, capable of neutralising the invading, invisible enemies. Sometimes these warriors play havoc with our own body by mistaking harmless substances such as pollen for enemies, thereby causing allergic reactions. Occasionally our defenders are routed and we catch a cold or get an infection. But for every successful penetration of our defense system, there are literally hundreds of repelled attacks. Our "vigilantes" are constantly on the alert, prepared to confront any foreign body filtrating through our defense system.

Our "vigilantes" or defender white cells arise in the bone marrow and spleen and fall into three groups. One kind are the **phagocytes**, which are the housekeepers, and two types of lymphocytes, called **T and B cells**. All share one common objective: recognize and destroy all "corpora aliena" or "foreign bodies." These highly specialised white blood cells, about one trillion strong, engage in millions of battle encounters against formidable opponents. These are the "Star Wars" of our body.

Let's depict a classical battle against the simplest and yet most devious enemy: the virus. As viruses begin to invade the body, the battle begins. The first defenders to arrive are the phagocytes, the house cleaners of the system. They are not choosy, thank God! Constantly alert, they roam through our bodies searching for anything that seems to be out of place. They waste no time, any invader they find is engulfed and consumed within seconds. Yes, they can cleanse lungs that have been blackened by smoking or other environmental pollutants, such as asbestos or silica. But, do not push your luck! There will come a time when the destruction of phagocytes will supercede the replenishment.

A special kind of phagocyte is the macrophage. The macrophage literally eats the enemy, digesting and metabolizing its materials. Macrophages and other phagocytes are produced in the bone marrow and are present throughout the bloodstream and tissues of the body. Phagocytes are especially abundant in the liver, an organ with unusual concentration of cellular debris, and in the lungs, where they cleanse the tissue of airborne pathogens and particles. When the macrophage attacks a virus, it plucks a special piece, called antigen, from this invader. This antigen is then displayed on its own cell surface like a captured war trophy. That trophy plays a critical role in the response of the fine machinery of the immune system. It will alert a highly classified kind of cell, the Helper T-cell, commander-in-chief of our immune system.

All our lives, millions of these Helper T-cells circulate in our bloodstream. This is truly a miracle of ingenuity. Among millions of these Helper T-cells, there is one that can read the antigen displayed on that macrophage and fit its receptor exactly into it. How did they become so well trained? The Helper T-cell training took place in the thymus, a gland located behind the breastbone above the heart. That is why they are named "T" cells: THYMUS-derived cells. This gland swells in size from birth to puberty and then begins to shrink. As the T-cells mature in the thymus, the strongest ones are selected to identify the antigens of any possible enemy, virus, bacteria or yeast cell. The ones with lesser powers of recognition die in the thymus. In view of the hundreds of millions of antigens nature creates, the thymus confronts a staggering task, because it must turn out T-cells that recognize each enemy. Even more mind-boggling is the fact that we have T-cells trained to identify artificial antigens created in the lab -- antigens the body never encountered in its entire existence. (The cellular migrations of lymphocytes after birth are rather complex. Significant numbers of these cells leave the thymus shortly after birth to settle in the lymph nodes and the spleen. On the other hand, a constant stream of bone-marrow precursors invades the thymus throughout life). (See Fig. # 1)

But let's go back to our battle plan! As we have seen, the T-cell binds to the macrophage and thus becomes activated. Once activated, Helper T-cells, begin to multiply. Their task is not to kill, as they carry no weapons. Rather, they are like the battlefield general, who sends urgent chemical signals to a small squadron of front soldiers -- the KILLER T-CELLS. There is only ONE message: MULTIPLY FAST! Killer T-cells are also trained to recognize one particular enemy, and once they receive the message from the Helper T-cells, this little squadron grows into an irresistible army. They either puncture the cell membranes of bacteria or destroy infected cells before the virus has time to multiply. Since the inside of the cells is the only place where the virus can replicate, the viral replication cycle is disrupted right there.

But the Helper T-cell calls on a second platoon of well-trained soldiers. They rush toward the spleen and lymph nodes and alert the paratroopers of the immune system: the B-CELLS. These cells are born in the bone marrow and migrate primarily to our lymph nodes. We only become aware of these bean-shaped capsules during infections, when they become swollen and sometimes painful to the touch, a sign that our immune systems are fighting back! The lymph nodes are widely distributed throughout the body and are normally less than one-half inch long. These lymph nodes are strategically placed at crossroads, which might be easily defendable outposts Compare it to an army commander placing his troops at mountain passes. During infections, lymphocytes trap the invaders in lymph nodes removing them from the bloodstream.

The B-cells function as small munitions factories, producing chemical weapons called antibodies. When the Killer T-cells puncture the membranes of the infected cells, the virus spills out where the antibodies of the B-cells can directly bind to the surface of the virus, preventing it from killing other cells. By sticking to the surface, these antibody molecules slow down the virus enough to make it an easier target -- as well as a more attractive one -- for phagocytes. Antibodies do not only neutralize; they also kill! They fit on the enemy's antigen like a key in a lock and col-

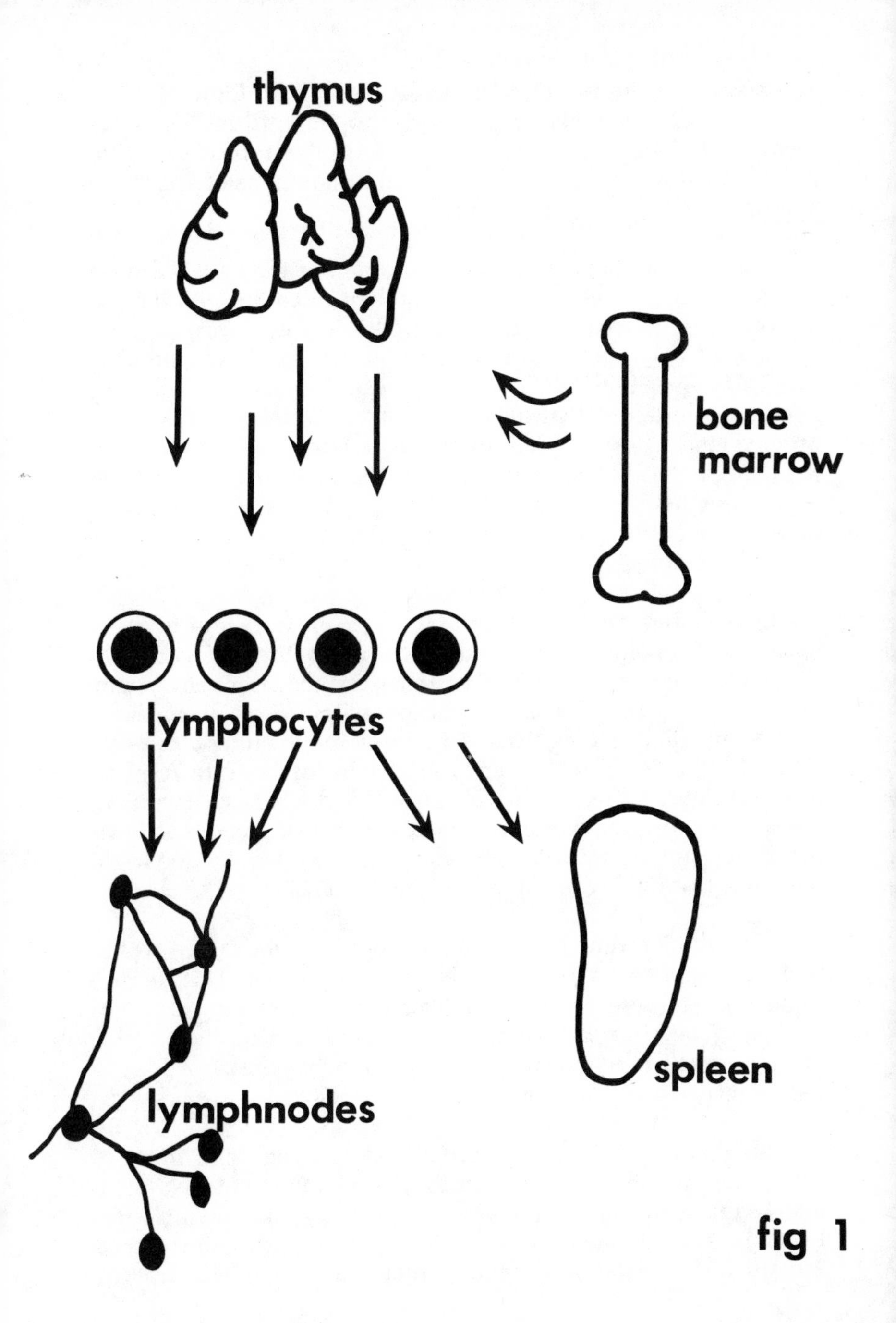

fig 1

lect substances in the bloodstream, called COMPLEMENT. The latter can detonate like a bomb, destroying the invader's cell membrane. Notice the reproductivity of these B-cells: at the peak of their operation, they can turn out thousands of antibodies a second, creating an awesome army.

Considering the size and sophistication of the body's armies, it is no small wonder that we win millions of battles. As the tide of these battles turns and the invaders are in retreat, a third member of the T-cell group takes command. These are the SUPPRESSOR T-CELLS, and they are ready to sign a truce by releasing substances that turn off B-cells and other T-cells. They order them to stop fighting: the battle is won. You can imagine the debacle that would result if we did not have enough of these suppressor T-cells. Our Killer T and Helper T-cells would continue to multiply out of control resulting in the eventual exhaustion of our immune system.

In the aftermath of these immune system wars, our army of house cleaners empties the battlefields of the litter of dead cells. The battles are over, but not forgotten by the immune system. Most of the T and B-cells will die off within days. But a large contingent will lead long lives and roam through our bodies as so-called MEMORY CELLS. They will enable the body to respond more quickly to subsequent infections. If and when we encounter the same enemy, the battle is over in a matter of seconds. The virus is recognized immediately and overwhelmed by the right kind of antibodies: we are immune. (Fig # 2a & b)

If everything ran as smoothly as described above, we would be in good shape. Alas, our T-cells are so diligent that they recognize even desirable cells transplanted from one person to another. They identify them as foreign and destroy them. This process, called rejection, can defeat a life-saving heart or kidney transplant and annihilate hours of surgical work.

Even more problematic is a devastating category of illnesses called autoimmune diseases. In these diseases the immune system attacks our own cells because they mistakenly take them for foreign bodies. Examples of these diseases are rheumatoid arthritis, MS, Systemic Lupus Erythematosus, Crohn's disease,

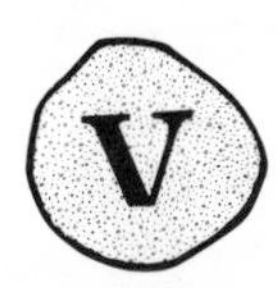

A virus is the cause of most common diseases. It is the simplest, yet the most devious enemy.

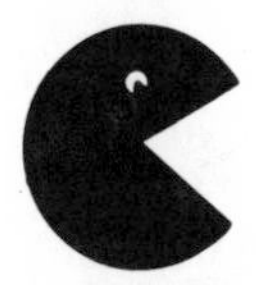

A Macrophage, the body's "Pac Man" roams throughout our body, consumes pollutants and other invaders at an incentive rate.

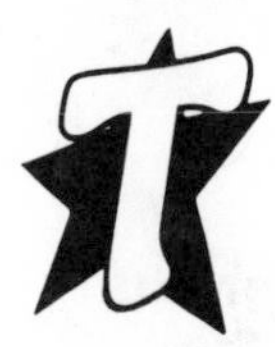

The T-Helper cell, the commander-in-chief of our immune system. The fine mechanism of our defense system depends on its ability to activate the other defender-cells.

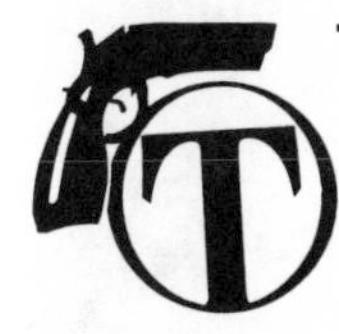

The T-Killer cell, activated by the T-Helper cell, has only one goal: destroy the enemy before it has time to multiply.

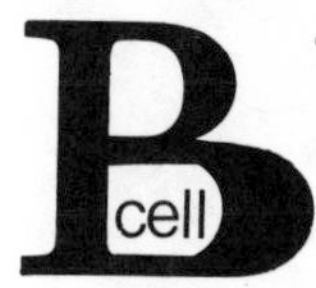

The B-cell, activated again by the T-Helper cell multiplies in the spleen and lymph nodes. They produce their weapons called antibodies.

fig. 2a

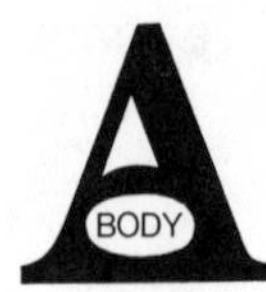

Antibodies, produced by B-cells, stick to the surface of viruses, slow them down, but are also able to kill viruses.

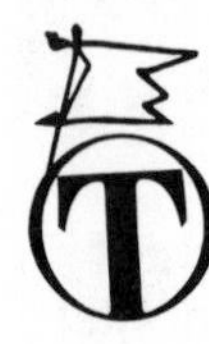

T-Suppressor cell will call the battle off when victory has been achieved. They tell the T-Killer cells to stop the fight.

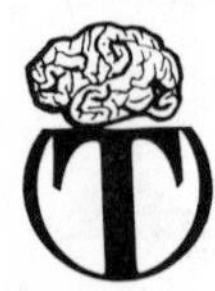

T-Memory cell stays in the body after the infection. It is trained to recognize the invasion of the same enemy in the future.

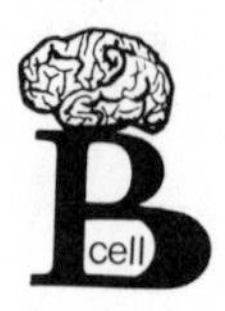

B-Memory cell has the same function as the T-Memory cell. It will produce antibodies, upon recognizing the same enemy.

2a continued

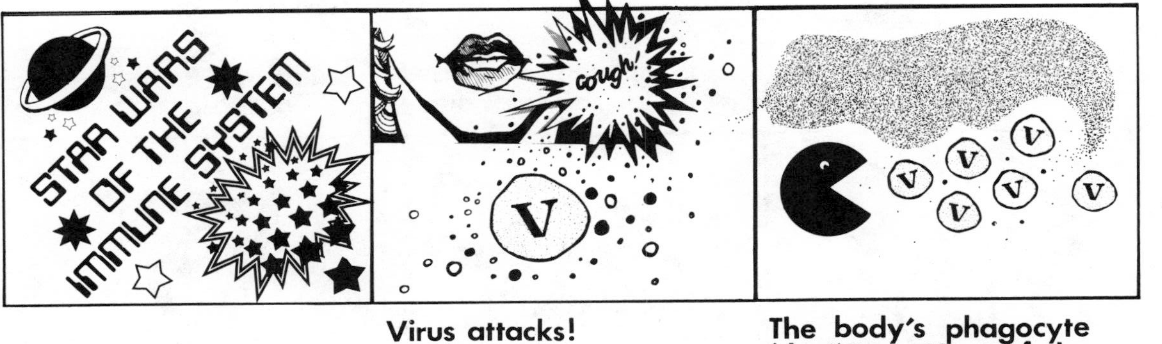

Virus attacks!

The body's phagocyte (the "Pac Man" of the immune system) attacks the viruses.

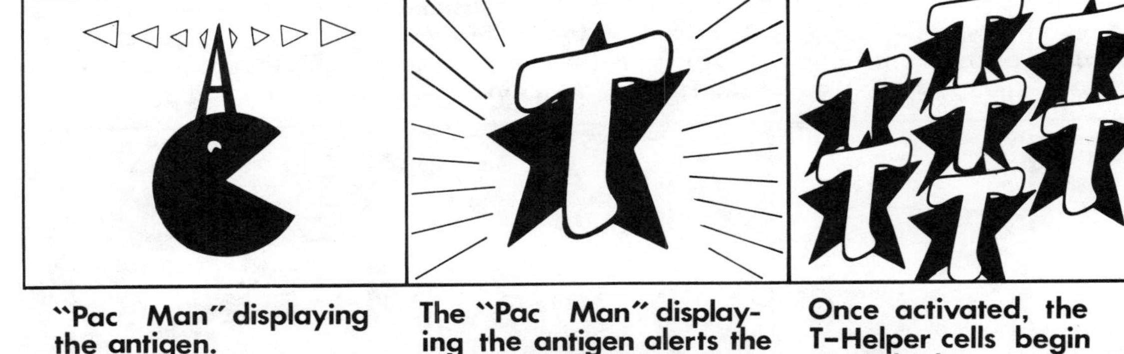

"Pac Man" displaying the antigen.

The "Pac Man" display-ing the antigen alerts the T-Helper cell. (Command-er-in-chief of our immune

Once activated, the T-Helper cells begin to multiply.

fig 2b

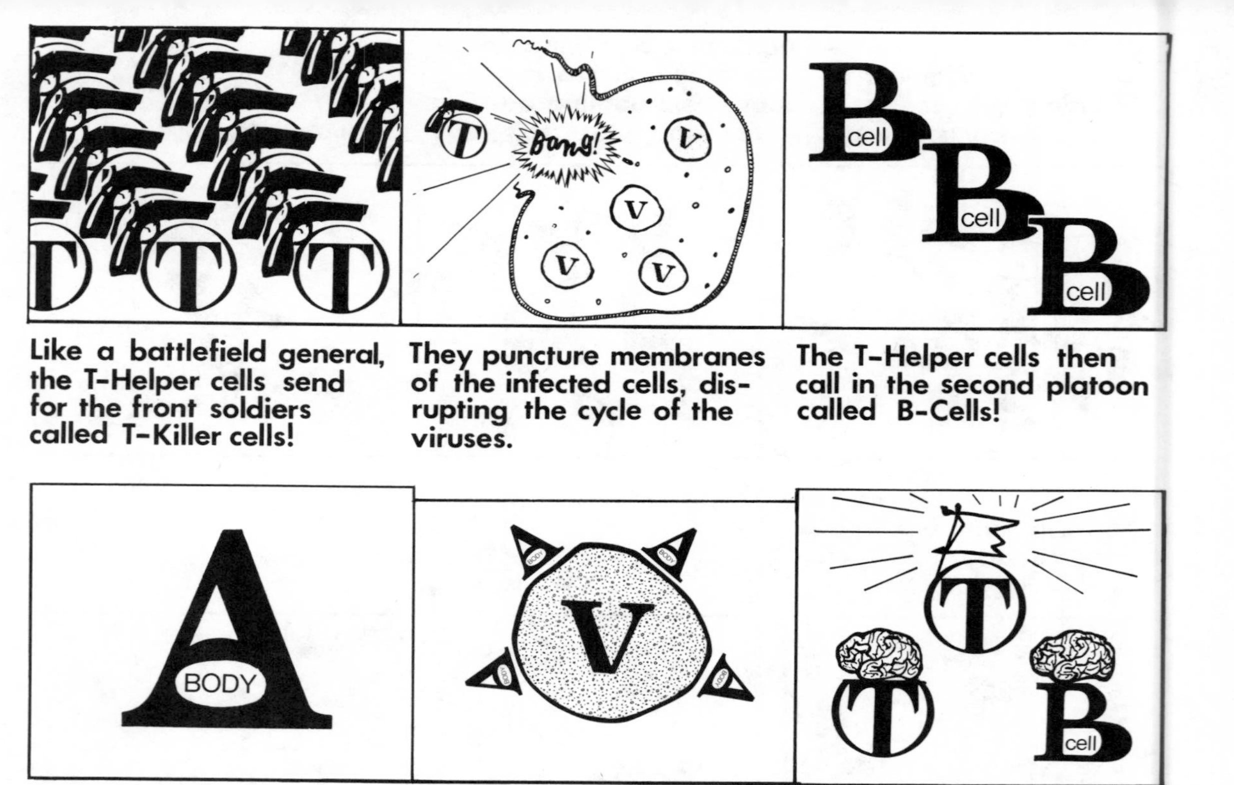

fig. 2b continued

ulcerative colitis and scleroderma. At this point, Western medicine does not have a remedy for these diseases except the administration of cortisone. Cortisone will suppress the activity of the immune system, which causes it to slow down its action. On the other hand, it means that we decrease our resistance to various infections, viral, bacterial, yeast..."The blessing of a false bishop," we used to call cortisone in our student days. This is understandable if you look at the initial euphoric action combined with the side effects after prolonged use, such as ulcers, osteoporosis, decreased resistance to infection, diabetes and Cushing's disease, to name just a few.

Moreover, this is not the only error of judgment that the immune system makes. It sometimes mounts battles against phantom enemies. Thousands of harmless substances -- pollen and dust -- cause allergic reactions in some 40 million Americans. The allergen itself is no threat. Most people are exposed to it without any consequence except for hay-fever sufferers, whose immune systems mistakenly recognize pollen as an enemy. The immediate reaction is a spill of potent chemicals, such as histamine, released by specialized mast cells. And our faithful T-cells make matters worse by ordering B-cells to produce more antibodies. So our sneezing spells, runny nose and tearing eyes are simply signs of an overreacting immune system.

Do we know everything about the immune system at this stage? Not at all. We know as little about the immune system now as Columbus knew about the Americas after his first trip. In other words, we have only seen the tip of the iceberg. Even with sophisticated tools like electronic microscopes, monoclonal antibodies and recombinant DNA, we are still unable to match the achievement of an English country physician who, 200 years ago and with no knowledge of the immune system, scored one of medicine's greatest triumphs. As with a lot of great inventions, Dr. Edward Jenners' findings were based on observations and a stroke of luck. He absolutely had no idea how it worked but he saw that people infected with the mild cowpox infection were protected against the far more serious smallpox infection. He therefore had the idea of infecting people with cowpox and eureka! It worked. People infected with cowpox were protected against smallpox. Of course, he could not know how incredibly lucky he was, for the cowpox resembles the smallpox so closely that the immune system cannot tell them apart. Hence, an army of memory T-cells, formed after being inoculated with the mild cowpox, encountered and neutralized the smallpox invaders of his patients.

So where will the new frontiers of immunology lead us? Waiting for advances in modern medicine to receive more information about the mysterious immune system is one option. However, I feel that ancient medicine has always had a better understanding about how the immune system may be affected by mind/body relation. Acupuncture, a 5000-year-old medicine, has always taken into account the mind and the body. I think this is something we miss in modern medicine: we do not let our mind relate to our heart, we keep it in our cranium, to achieve the ultimate in reasoning. It might be useful to go back 5000 years in history and see what the wise Chinese medical men thought about the immune system.

If there is one misunderstanding about acupuncture in our Western world, it is the thought that acupuncture only relieves pain. In other words, it is purely symptomatic but does not effect a cure, and that using acupuncture for anything else but "pain" conditions is a laughable attempt to imitate Western medicine. I don't know who started this nonsense, and I really don't care. All I know is that it is a great insult to one of the most promising arts of medicine known. It is enough to point out its long survival to indicate that acupuncture is more than just a fad. Ancient Chinese printing and the famous Chinese arts (pottery and painting) also were at unmatched heights. It is only fitting that Chinese medicine should coincide with the eminence of the whole culture. Acupuncture laws were the result of thousands of years of observation. For the Chinese, it was simple: nature and mankind cause the disease, and nature has the cure for it. According to the Chinese, there were 10 organs, coupled to each other in what they call "the Yin-Yang" relationship. It is not my intent to elaborate on the details of acupuncture. Rather, I will illustrate in this text how it relates to the Chinese concept of "Immunity." It is my strong belief that we can learn from this old art to assist in overcoming the cluster of immune-suppressed diseases that have afflicted us.

The organs, according to the Chinese, had several well-defined functions. The one that is important to us here is the spleen-pancreas organ. For the Chinese this was one organ, while in our Western world, the spleen and pancreas are considered two separate, independently-functioning organs. I believe that we have not unlocked all the secrets of cooperation between these two organs, and this fact may prove to be very important in combatting the immune-suppressed diseases. We do not think much of the spleen as an organ in Western medicine. Don't we remove the spleen easily in trauma when it is ruptured, without apparent consequences? However, I do not know of any study done to see if these victims did not suffer a higher incidence of immune-suppressed diseases. I base this belief on the known functions of the spleen in acupuncture.

In the first place, the spleen is the most important organ in the transformation and transportation of food. In other words, lack of energy in this organ leads to malabsorption and under-nutrition, certainly not a good boost for the immune system. However, a second, more important, function is the production of the white blood cells, the key-defenders of our immune system. Hence, lack of energy in the spleen-pancreas may result in a suppressed immune system. The various causes of this decreased energy may contribute to a suppressed immune system. Let us examine these causes and see what we can learn.

The Chinese believed that any cause of disease can be reduced to four main groups:

HEREDITARY FACTORS

FOOD

EMOTIONS

EXTERNAL FACTORS

By observing the laws of acupuncture and taking into consideration these four causal groups, we can begin to get an understanding as to what went wrong with our immune systems.

2. HOW DID WE ARRIVE AT THE BREAKDOWN OF OUR IMMUNE SYSTEMS AT THIS TIME IN OUR HISTORY?

A. HERIDIDARY FACTORS

Hereditary factors are important, and we cannot change them, of course, but we must be aware of the dangers we incur if we neglect to protect ourselves. How many times will patients recognize that their parents went through the same symptom complex as they and accepted it like helpless victims at the time, since clear diagnosis was impossible. If a person knows he risks a certain disease because the incidence is high in his family, taking the three other factors into account (food, emotions and external factors) will help to avoid the same disease. What this means for our immune system is that hereditary diseases of the spleen and pancreas, such as diabetes, certain purpuras or bleeding diseases and hypoglycemia, will affect the strength of the immune system more than is generally thought.

The list of hereditary diseases is an extensive one, and a complete description of them is beyond the scope of this book. However, because of its prevalence and its devastating effect on people, depressive illness will be considered here.

DEPRESSION

It chills the heart and saps the will even to get out of bed. It paralyses. Victims often experience a terrifying loneliness, a sense of being "outside" of themselves. There is only cold, inside and outside. The sun seems to have lost its normal warmth. Every move takes an enormous effort, like a nightmare in slow motion. It is not possible to think about joy in life; there is no joy in life. Not surprisingly, many victims are driven to take their own lives, accounting for about 60% of all suicides. So high is the incidence of depression that it is called "the common cold" of mental illness. Amazingly enough, with the help that is available, only 20% seek help. They lose jobs, friends, family and sometimes simply wait for the final escape: death. What is more disturbing, depression is on the rise among young people. Reasonable speculations have been made as to the cause: disruption of family ties, drug abuse, alcoholism. But I have no doubt that the high incidence of depression is also the result of changes in nutrition (mass sugar consumption) and the spread of viral (EBV) or yeast (Candida) infections. This viewpoint is not widely accepted in the medical community, but I have seen evidence of it time and time again. Our young people are the first-line victims of these changes, and we older adults have a hard time understanding this situation.

Researchers are gaining new insights as to why some people are more susceptible than others. The most exciting recent finding is the identification of a genetic link to manic depression or a so-called bi-polar form of the disorder. It is characterized by sharp mood swings, instead of the continuous lows, typical of depression. It was known for some time that this disease ran in families; but the discovery provides for the first time a clear indication that a predisposition may be passed along through generations. Recently a team of scientists at Miami University's School of Medicine studied an 81-member Amish family in Pennsylvania, interviewing members and sampling their blood for genetic material. Nearly 80% of the subjects with a certain marker on one of the 46 human chromosomes had manic depression. According to the researchers, inheriting the marker predisposes them to manic depression. I think it would be very helpful to study concurrently their patterns in diet, the environments they live in and the factors they have in common. Since they all belong to the same family, they inevitably will have many similar habits. Those 20% not affected might give us the clue: it would be interesting to see if they differ at all in their lifestyles.

How do people deal with depression? Some will pretend that there is no problem. Others will treat the condition by running miles every day. This is not such a bad idea, since the running, especially long-distance, will release the natural endorphins, creating a sense of well-being. Of course, let's not forget that during their "lows", these people will not "move from their chairs," let alone run for miles. Others will take their refuge in medications. There are at least some remedies available, which work to varying degrees in different people. Most of the time it is a search for the patient and the doctor to find the right doses.

Available drugs are mentioned in Table # 1.

B. THE FOOD CONNECTION

Before dealing with current wisdom, let's see what the Chinese thought about food and immunity. As previously indicated, the organ we have to focus on is the spleen-pancreas. The Chinese knew that the taste of food was important in keeping an organ in balance. If there is too much intake of a taste, the organ energy decreases; if there is too little, the result is the same, the organ energy is not boosted. In other words, organs need the taste of food in a certain strength to keep their energy maintained. Through extensive observation, the Chinese knew exactly which type of taste relates to which organ. The one belonging to the spleen-pancreas, thus important to the immune system, is the sweet taste. The connection of the other tastes with their organs is shown in the figure below. (See Fig.# 3)

Let's examine the sweet taste. As you will notice, I do not talk about calorie content or sugar. And that's where we have made a major mistake in our modern nutrition. Preoccupied with weight gain, smart business people have introduced NUTRASWEET, claiming that it has no calories but -- and here comes the clue -- it is about TWO HUNDRED TIMES SWEETER than white sugar. NUTRASWEET swiftly received a clean bill of health from the FDA in 1981, and a major enemy of the immune system invaded our bodies. Name one soft drink company that has not introduced NUTRASWEET in its products. The consequences are disastrous: The energy in the spleen-pancreas decreases dramatically, or in other words, the immune system is depressed each time we introduce NUTRASWEET. NUTRASWEET is derived from aspartame (a man-made chemical); EQUAL and SWEET-AND-LOW are other brand names for similar sweeteners. And that's not all. That it contains fewer calories, therefore inducing weight loss, is absolutely untrue. As you already can guess from the discussion about the spleen-pancreas, its transformation function will be hampered by the excessive quantity of sweet taste. In other words, your digestive capacities decrease each time you ingest aspartame. The final result is weight gain. It would be very interesting to do a double-blind study, one group taking water or even vegetable juices, the other Nutrasweet drinks and

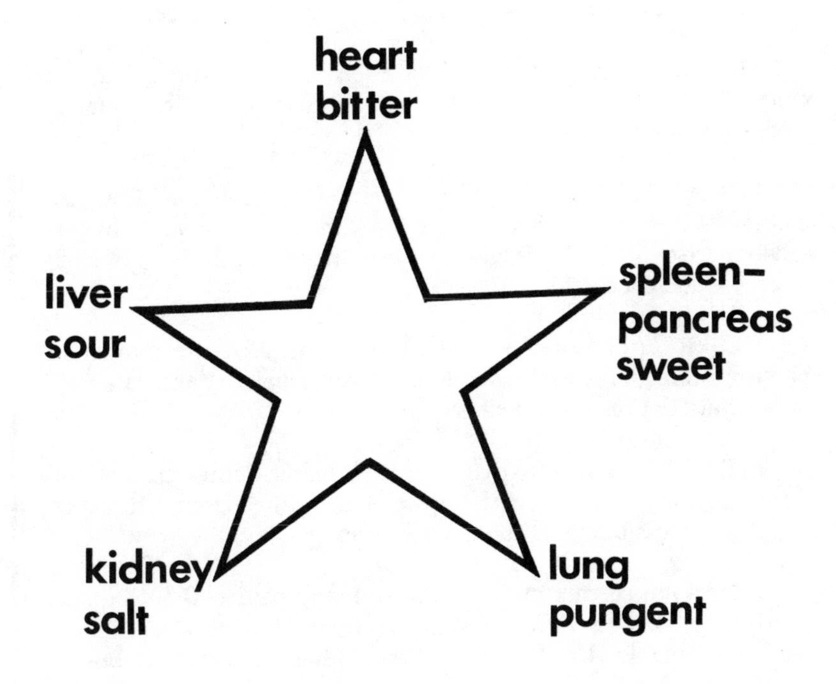
heart
bitter
spleen-
pancreas
sweet
lung
pungent
kidney
salt
liver
sour

Fig 3

DRUG TREATMENT (Table # 1)

Many patients take one of these drugs to control depression:

ELAVIL: a tricyclic derivative -- a class of drugs that includes Tofranil, Vivactil, Norpramin. Possible side effects: drowsiness, nausea, dry mouth.

PARNATE: a MAO (Mono-Amino-Oxydase) inhibitor. Includes Marplan. Possible dangers: seizures, rash and hypertensive crises with the intake of tyramine-containing foods such as cheese and chocolate.

DESYREL: one of the newer drugs, but also with danger of persistent erection (rare), impotence, liver problems and fatigue -- not what a depressed patient needs.

LITHIUM: first line drug for the manic-depressed patient. Excess dosage, however, is associated with extreme toxicity, therefore necessitating frequent blood tests.

It does not seem a tragedy that so many people should go on bearing the burden of misery that depression inflicts when help is readily available. Up to now, research has provided at best a clouded window on its origins.

see which group actually loses weight. I would bet all my money on the outcome: NUTRASWEET would be the loser.

Speaking of soft drinks, let's examine some hard facts about them. Americans today are drinking more soda pop than they are plain water. Let that sink in for a moment. The average American consumes more soft drinks in a year than water. Documentation for this statistic comes from a trade publication called: "Beverage Industry." Here are the figures: In 1986, Americans drank 42 gallons of soft drinks per capita. They drank 41 gallons of water. This seems to be the culmination of a trend that has been forming for 20 years. Consumption of water has been going down steadily, while the use of soft drinks has risen dramatically. The only question was when soft-drink consumption would surpass water. It has finally happened. To show how dramatic this change has been, in 1964 the per capita consumption of water was 72 gallons a year; the per capita consumption of soft drinks was 17 gallons a year.

Why these changes? The Baby Boom Generation is partly to blame. It was raised on soft drinks. People do not spend as much time at home as they used to, and soft drink machines are everywhere. Every business location and office has a vending machine. There are about two million in the U.S. at the moment. Another reason for this overconsumption of soft drinks is the fact that soft drink companies spend a lot more money on advertising, and there is no advertising for plain water. The advertising makes soft drinks seem fashionable, like the socially-correct thing to do. It is the beverage that you consume when you fall in love, when you meet friends, etc. Advertising has almost made the 12-ounce soft drink container part of the human hand. This may be another reason for our decreasing health status: the common glass of water is an endangered species.

But is there a "natural" alternative that can satisfy our sweet tooth? Unfortunately, no such sweetener exists (except maybe fruit juices). We should keep in mind that only small quantities of sweetener are necessary to maintain health. On the other hand, excessive sugar intake has been linked to arthritis, hypertension, diabetes, dental decay and equally important, depression and fatigue. Americans today consume over fifteen times the amount of sugar they did 100 years ago.

All sweeteners are concentrated simple sugars and as such can not be considered whole foods. Natural sweeteners have many of the same effects on the body as white sugar. If we eat whole foods, the vitamins, minerals and enzymes present will allow smooth metabolism of the sugars contained therein. The best way for the body to take in sugar is through the digestion of complex carbohydrates: the starch from grains, vegetables and fruits are digested slowly, releasing sugar in the blood gradually. This prevents the insulin overload and adrenal exhaustion that accompanies the ingestion of concentrated simple sugars. But the message is clear: stay away from sweets (except fruits) to preserve your digestive powers and general health.

The sweet taste was not the only connection the Chinese made with the immune system. There is another enemy of the spleen-pancreas: **Dampness**, and particularly, **Cold-Dampness**. Through observation, the Chinese knew that **raw** and cold foods transform in the spleen into Heat-Dampness, thus decreasing its transforming capacities. It upsets a lot of people when I mention this, since we think about the rich enzyme content present in raw food. However, anybody who has suffered from any malabsorption syndrome has experienced difficulty digesting raw foods, especially vegetables. To protect the strength of our spleen and our immune system, we should cook, steam or stir-fry our vegetables.

Let's return to modern times and see what "progress" we have made. A great many health officials and doctors still think we have the best food supply in the world and that the intake of vitamins is unfounded, ridiculous and simply a fad. Look at some recent headlines in magazines and newspapers: "U.S. Food Safety Doubted;" "Improper Use of Equipment Leads to Tainted Poultry;" "FDA Plans to Stop Widespread Use of Antibiotics in Stock Food;" "Adding Up Additives: a Difficult Job, But It Must be Done;" "What Price for Clean, Safe Food?" "Experts Say that the Consumer Would be Surprised at All that Slips In;" "Disturbing Study on Store Meats;" "Deceptive Ads are Now O.K.;" "Children's Behavior Affected by Food Intake." I could go on ad infinitum. These are just a few samples I found in medical magazines and the lay press in the past year. Do you think I am exaggerating? In fact the problem is much worse and has inevitably contributed to many diseases.

We can start with the routine addition of antibiotics to the feed of chickens, cows and pigs. Many patients try to convert to vegetarianism. This is not an unusual reaction, because they see little good in these antibiotics and the potential for harm. Although people who raise cows or pigs insist that they must use antibiotics to prevent infections and promote growth, knowledgeable critics are now "blowing the whistle" on them and raising the "red flag."

Authorities in England put a stop to adding low doses of antibiotics to the feed of livestock and poultry in 1971. So did a number of other countries in Europe. The FDA recommended a similar ban in 1977. However, Congress said "No," maintaining that more data was needed to make certain that tetracyclines added to the animal food posed a serious threat to the nation's health.

The gravest threat is that regular feeding of antibiotics may produce bacteria resistant to it and lead to their multiplication in the flesh of the animal. The problem gets worse when people ingest antibiotics, thus killing off their healthy intestinal bacteria and allowing the overgrowth of yeast cells. So there is a good chance that tonight's dinner has been laced with the wonder drugs developed after World War II to fight diseases from tonsillitis to gonorrhea. Antibiotics are so prevalent today as to be on the verge of losing their effectiveness against some new strains of bacteria that have grown resistant to the drugs. Moreover, the resistance to antibiotics already found in animals is capable of being transferred to human beings.

The consequences are obvious: it is a serious risk to human health; with the recent emergence of resistant strains of bacteria causing pneumonia, meningitis and venereal disease, the threat becomes formidable indeed. A study done in the U.S. in 1982 and published in the New England Journal of Medicine showed that bits of genes that cause resistance may be capable of transferring their properties to bacteria strains that attack only humans and may be a major part of the growing problem of antibiotic resistance among people. These studies establish that resistant animal bacteria and human bacteria are interconnected. The investigation team studied salmonella bacteria, which can cause lethal disease in cattle and are among the most common causes of food-poisoning in humans.

Of course, all these claims will provoke reactions from industry spokesmen, who want more "hard evidence." Just as we should wait for a nuclear power plant to explode in order to establish that it is wise to regulate them! How much longer do we have to wait? Right now we have epidemics of diseases linked to food intake, although antibiotics obviously are not the only culprits.

As if the legal additives weren't bad enough, a study by government inspectors indicates that 14% of the dressed meat and poultry sold in supermarkets may contain illegal residues of drugs, pesticides or other contaminants. The Department of Agriculture had to admit that at this time they "don't have the scientific knowledge or technological skills to ensure that no contaminated meat or poultry reaches the market."

A tabulation of all the additives in food is another difficult job. It is difficult -- maybe impossible -- to avoid these additives entirely, because we do have to eat. What can we do? The first thing is to find out which ones are really dangerous and avoid those 100% of the time. When parents tell me this is impossible with children, I tell them about all the mothers I know who love their children so much that they are determined to win this battle. Their kids don't get any food with harmful additives at home and are so well-conditioned that when they leave home, they choose not to eat them. Of course, it means that the parents have to set the example, and therein lies the difficulty.

There is a poster entitled "Chemical Cuisine" that tells you which of the most often-encountered additives are dangerous and which ones appear to be safe. (If you want this wall poster, write to CSPI, P.O. Box 3099, Washington, D.C. 20010). Below are some of those on the list to avoid. Artificial coloring heads the list. It certainly is illogical to make the fattening foods, which we should avoid in the first place, even more attractive by coloring them brightly and enhancing the taste with artificial flavors. Simply avoid all artificially-colored foods, especially the worst ones: Blue Nos. 1 and 2; Green # 3; Orange B; Red # 3; Red # 40; Yellow # 5; and Citrus Red # 2, which is used to dye the skin of some Florida oranges.

Other additives to avoid are artificial flavorings: BVO found in soft drinks; BHT, found in cereals, chewing gum, and potato chips; and nitrites and nitrates, found in almost all processed meats, bacon, sausages and smoked fish. The best thing to do is to stay with natural, unprocessed foods, and the safer you are likely to be.

If the above facts have not worried you yet, listen to this. In March 1987, a segment on the popular CBS Newsmagazine "60 Minutes" drew the attention of the public toward bacteria-tainted poultry. "America's food-safety system has broken down, and consumers are at high risk from contaminated poultry," inspectors from the U.S. Department of Agriculture claimed in an open letter to the Secretary of Agriculture. Bacteria-tainted poultry and food poisoning cases have risen dramatically because the equipment used to mass-produce poultry fosters contamination. The bacteria levels are a direct result of the reckless use of new technologies. Those include eviscerating machines that rip open the intestines and spread manure and undigested feed through the carcass, and a washing process that ends by bathing the already soiled birds in chilled tanks, so filthy that inspectors refer to them as fecal soup.

What is the answer of USDA officials? They defend the system stating that improvements would be costly and affect supermarket prices. So to save a dime, they would rather ruin our health, which will cost us billions of dollars in medical care, to say nothing of the misery it will bring families because of disease that could have been easily prevented. Costly indeed: to our health! The USDA has acknowledged that nearly 40 percent of the poultry sold in the United States is contaminated with Salmonella, a bacteria that can be fatal and is among the most common causes of food poisoning. Because of the high cost of overhauling the food inspection system (and its impact on consumer prices) USDA officials favor gradual changes in which poultry producers would clean up their plants. I do not agree at all with this policy! I'd rather pay a little more with the knowledge that I am eating safe food. Many of my patients, after viewing "60 Minutes," refused to eat chicken at all! We all should boycott unsafe food, our very lives may depend on it.

Looking at the past thirty years, what are the major changes in our diet that have resulted in the diet-related diseases we now struggle with? I think these changes were triggered by the combination of the consumers' desire for convenience and manufacturers' competitiveness. With the higher cost of living and an increased desire for luxury, busy people require quickly prepared, palatable and rather inexpensive food. Food chemists responded to these needs, adding colorings, preservatives and flavorings, creating overnight a new era in the food industry. The supermarket was born.

We can see that those dietary changes are enormous. First, we now consume an increasing amount of fat. Indeed, by feeding animals corn to make the meat more tender, the fat content is twice as much as in meat from range-fed animals. As if that were not bad enough, we increase the intake of the wrong fats. At the beginning of this century, our diets contained mainly Omega-3 fatty acids (in the form of fish). They have been found to be extremely important in avoiding heart disease. Today, however, we use 95% of Omega-6 fats (pork, fried foods, chips) versus 5% Omega-3 fats. Omega-3 fats produce hormone-like substances (Prostaglandins), important to the immune system and proper cell activity.

Another major change is the reduced intake of dietary fiber. No wonder constipation is an almost accepted symptom in our society. Initially fiber was defined as being the roughage of plants left after the digestive process. Recently crude fibers include some substances such as pectins, gums and mucilages found in many fruits. They form viscous solutions that soften the stool and may favorably prolong the nutrient transport time in the gastrointestinal tract. Scientists became aware of the crucial role of fiber in the diet through studies of native Japanese who, upon arriving in Hawaii, adopted the low-fiber, high-fat Western diet. They suddenly developed heart and intestinal diseases previously unknown to them, including appendicitis, colon cancer, diabetes, myocardial infarction and obesity. Americans have diets that are abnormally low in fiber. We should increase our intake to 30 grams of fiber a day, depending on our size (large individuals should consume more).

To make matters worse, the processing of whole grains to white-flour products removes many of the trace minerals, such as copper, zinc, chromium, and selenium, all of which we already consume less in our diets. Intensive modern agricultural methods have robbed the soil of trace elements, essential human nutrients.

We almost forgot enemy number one: increased intake of sugar. One of the consequences is a decreased amount of copper, leading to elevated cholesterol and increased risk of arteriosclerosis.

Are you still convinced that we have the best food in the world? Do you still think that those major dietary changes are not contributing to disease? Only naive people can hold this opinion.

C. EXTERIOR FACTORS

It is amazing, again, to see how much further Chinese medicine was evolved in the knowledge of the relationship of exterior factors and pathogenesis of disease. In all the exterior factors, one factor, mostly still neglected in our modern medicine, stood out: the climate factor. The Chinese knew exactly what climate factor influenced what organ in a negative way. Dampness, as mentioned above, is the worst factor for our immune system, since it decreases the strength in the spleen-pancreas organ. The same is true of dampness combined either with heat or cold. The combination is, in fact, even more devastating to the spleen. But other organs have their own climatic enemy. The lung (attention, asthma sufferers), decreases in strength in dryness, so the desert will not always favor patients with lung-related diseases. That is also why those patients suffer mostly in the fall, since this is the season of the lung, with maximum exposure to Dryness. The liver -- and liver patients -- are bothered by the wind or, as the Chinese called it, "fong." There is a good reason for this name. Fong means actually a lot more than Wind. It is everything that is brought by the wind: pollen (allergies), parasites and viruses.

Another climatic factor well known to arthritis sufferers is cold. Cold will decrease the energy in the kidney and adversely affect the bones. Now we come to the last "vicious factor", as the Chinese called it, heat. Heat suppresses the heart organ, and therefore, heart sufferers should avoid extreme heat exposure. I mean not only desert climates but also saunas and steam baths. The relationship between climate factors and organs is illustrated in Fig.# 4.

I would hope that modern medicine will start recognizing these factors and use them to our benefit: "cold conditions," such as arthritis and cancer, should be treated with Heat; "hot conditions," such as infections, inflammations and soft tissue traumas, with cold; "dry conditions," such as asthma or laryngitis, with Dampness, and so on. Besides the climate factor, other "Exterior Factors" are equally important and are becoming some of the gravest threats to our existence:

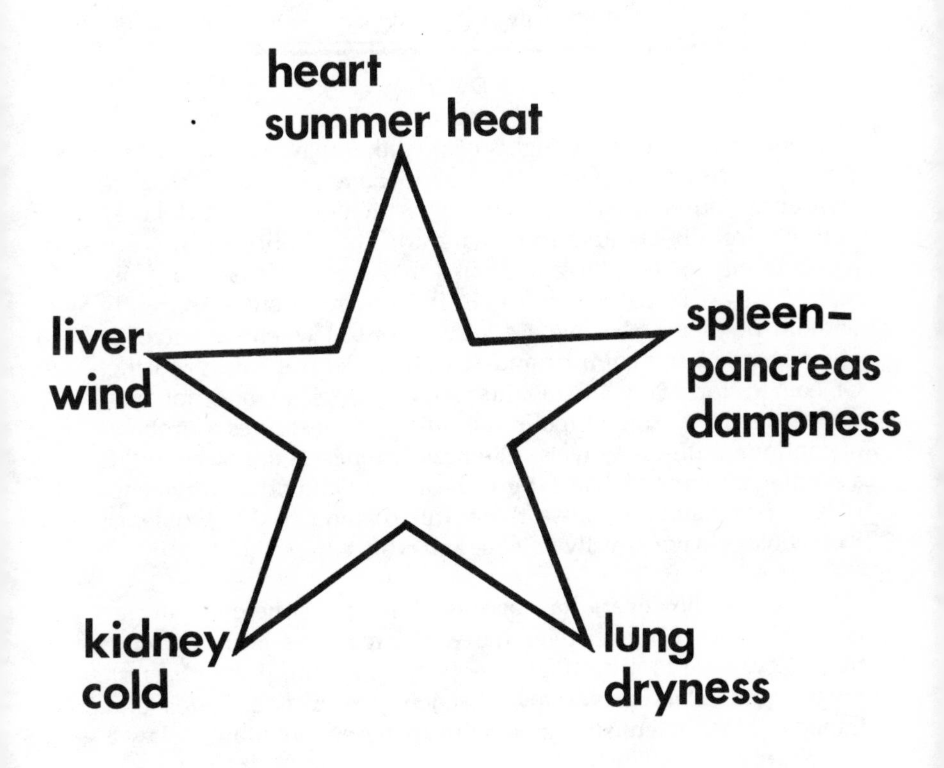
heart
summer heat
liver
wind
spleen-
pancreas
dampness
kidney
cold
lung
dryness

Fig 4

PESTICIDES IN SOIL AND AIR

POLLUTION OF OUR DRINKING WATER
LAKES AND RIVERS

EXPOSURE TO CIGARETTE SMOKE

MEDICATIONS

LIFE-STYLE CHANGES

1. PESTICIDES IN SOIL AND AIR

One of the greatest dangers of pollution may well be that we shall tolerate levels of it so low as to have no acute nuisance awareness, but sufficiently high, nevertheless, to cause delayed pathological effects and to downgrade the quality of life. For those living in the smog area of Los Angeles, this is a daily reality. We are so used to living in this environment, apparently without problems, that we are very surprised when we travel to other areas of the country and see our "allergies" disappearing. Of course, for many inhabitants of Los Angeles smog not only causes disease at some time in the future, it constitutes a problem of continuing illness as well. Often these illnesses are observed as a set of symptoms such as fatigue, headaches and other very generalized complaints. Because these are common health problems, their etiology is not directly obvious and is often missed.

The air, however, has become "an atmosphere of uncertainty." Stories from all over the world reach us with alarming frequency. Forests are afflicted not only in Central and Eastern Europe but also in Norway, Sweden, the United States and Canada. Most scientists agree that air-borne pollutants play a significant role in killing trees.

In other areas of the U.S.A. dirty air is held even more culpable. In Los Angeles we see that spectacular vistas are fading behind an aerosol haze. Pollutants resulting from automobile emissions annually reduce crop yields significantly, sometimes by as much as 20%, as in the soybean harvest for example.

What is not known about air pollution may be even more distressing. Thousands of commercial compounds enter our environment each year. Some are proven cancer-causing substances, and many more are suspected of being so. Yet only eight are listed as hazardous and are regulated at their source by the U.S. Environmental Protection Agency (EPA).

The Black Forest in West Germany was one of the most beautiful of its kind. However, now the needles of firs, spruces, and pines are turning yellow and falling off, leaving thin, scruffy crowns. Among the possible causes: oxides of sulfur and nitrogen from distant power plants and factories, nitrogen oxides from motor vehicles, and ozone from the interaction of air-borne chemicals in sunlight. And don't fool yourself: what happens there is commonplace here. These pollutants may also acidify the soil, destroying organisms necessary to the nutrient cycle, as well as injuring the trees' fine root systems. Weakened trees become more vulnerable to drought, insects and fungi. There is little reason for optimism.

As damage from our aerial "soup" concerns us more and more, an alarmed public clamors for answers and action. Both are slow in coming. Take, for example, the Carcinogen Assesssment Group, an arm of EPA. It was formed in 1976 to determine what chemical substances pose high cancer risks. Data on about only 200 commercial substances released in the air have been reviewed. Research is simply too expensive, and funding is totally inadequate. When we talk about an aerial "soup", the word is well chosen. Rarely does a city suffer from just a few air pollutants. Most cities generate a complex brew. Some chemicals are emitted directly from identifiable sources (see Table # 2); others are formed indirectly through photochemical reactions in the air (see Table # 3).

Table # 2

As (Arsenic): from coal and oil furnaces; long-time exposure causes lung and skin cancer.

CO (Carbon Monoxide): from motor vehicles, coal and oil furnaces, smelters, steel plants: starves the body of oxygen since the CO binds to the Hemoglobin; damages the heart.

CD (Cadmium): from smelters, burning waste, coal and oil furnaces; long-time exposure damages kidneys and lungs, weakens bones.

Ni (Nickel): from smelters, coal and oil furnaces; exposure may cause lung cancer.

NO (Nitric Oxide): from motor vehicles, coal and oil furnaces; readily oxidizes to NO2.

Mn (Manganese): from steel plants and power plants; long-time exposure may contribute to Parkinson's disease.

H2S (Hydrogen Sulfide): from refineries, sewage treatment plants, pulp mills; causes nausea and irritated eyes.

HCL (Hydrogen Chloride): from incinerators; irritates eyes and lungs.

Table # 3

NO2 (Nitrogen Dioxide): formed in sunlight from NO; produces ozone; causes bronchitis and lowers resistance to viral infections.

O3 (ozone): formed in sunlight from nitrogen oxides and hydrocarbons; irritates eyes and aggravates asthma and Chronic Obstructive Pulmonary Disease.

HNO3 (Nitric Acid): formed from NO2, is a major component of acid rain; causes respiratory ailments.

OH (Hydroxyl Radical): formed in sunlight from hydrocarbons and nitrogen oxides; reacts with other gases to form acid droplets.

Such chemical increases can be accommodated somehow, over time. However, the current overloading has the potential to alter life on this planet. And physically, our bodies already show the stress. Take lead, for example. Most of us are exposed through paint, plumbing, and principally automobile exhaust, despite a reduction in the lead content in gasoline. Although lead levels have been decreased in the U.S. over the last decade, excess lead in the human body can raise blood pressure. Decreasing everybody's lead levels by a third result in considerably fewer heart attacks over a decade.

And who can forget Chernobyl, the most dramatic example of man's concentrated effluents, posing far more danger than anything in nature? It will take many years before we even can assess the damage this catastrophe has brought down upon humanity.

Perhaps the most controversial environmental issue of the decade is acid rain, but that, too, is clouded in mystery. We are still in the early stages of understanding the full effects on an atmosphere acidified by burning fossil fuels. We need years of research in order to really grasp the problem. Acid rain was a primary topic at the April '87 summit between President Reagan and Canadian Prime Minister Brian Mulroney. Acid rain bills are being debated in Congress. New studies further detail its insidious effects. Yet public officials still refuse to take the big step toward solving the problem: curbing the emissions that cause acid rain.

The U.S.-Canada summit was a whitewash. Mulroney wanted an agreement, which he could not get, that would have placed limits on sulfur and nitrogen oxide emissions from U.S. plants. It is estimated that more than half of the acid rain falling on Canada comes from U.S. sources, not a very kind present to a friendly neighbor. Reagan sought to appease Mulroney while not deviating from his own long-held position that we don't know enough about acid rain to set such limits. Still holding on to his position in '88, President Reagan's actions or non-actions caused a strain in his longtime relationship with Mulroney. The problem is, resolutions to undertake "acid rain projects" generally translates into "more studies," not more action.

However, more studies are hardly necessary to show that action is necessary. Recent estimates by the Federal Office of Toxology Assessment say some 50,000 Americans may die prematurely each year from diseases caused or exacerbated by air-borne sulfates. New studies indicate that acid rain damages corn and leaches insecticides from the fields, causing farmers to spend more on chemicals. An EPA study estimates that each year acid precipitation causes some $5 billion in damage to buildings in the states east of the Mississippi River.

Another EPA study indicates that thousands of lakes in the U.S. are acid-rain sensitive. More bad news: New York State decided to permit Orange and Rockland Utilities, Inc. to start burning coal instead of natural gas at two units of its plant north of Manhattan. The plant could emit as much as 15,000 tons of sulfur dioxide a year, which would worsen the acid-rain problem even in the neighboring states.

How long have we had acid rain? Probably since the first rainfall. Volcanic eruptions and forest fires can produce sulfur or nitrogen compounds. However, as usual, nature preserves nature and keeps an excellent balance. It was mankind that changed this natural cycle begun with the clouds of coal smoke, that signal the start of the industrial revolution. Today a large coal-fired power plant in a single year can emit as much sulfur dioxide as was blown out by the 1980 eruption of Mount St. Helens in Washington State -- some 400,000 tons.

The total amounts of SO2 and NO that mankind releases are staggering. Canada, the U.S. and Europe together are responsible for the emission of 100 million tons of SO2 into the atmosphere a year. The economic surge that began with World War II brought increasing use of fossil fuels, and a corresponding increase in pollutants. Nevertheless, experts acknowledge that much remains to be learned about acid rain, even such basic questions as where exactly the specific sources of acid-causing pollutants are.

The reaction of soils to acid decomposition understandably stirs wide concern, for these are critical ecosystems, supporting the plants and animals that give us food, fiber, and forest products. How dim is the future? If acid deposition continues unabated, tracts of sensitive soils may slowly decline in fertility until their productivity fails. It is only a matter of time before we are forced to do something. Today's acid rain is only the beginning.

"Let's move to a deserted island," I hear you say, "just to escape this acid rain." I hate to disappoint you. SO2 and NO, along with other combustion products, climb skyward. There they circulate with the great air masses that form our weather systems. Their flight may last for hours, or days and take them thousands of miles. Because of these long journeys, acid deposition does not respect state or geographical boundaries. No effective solution to acid rain will be found as long as public officials refuse to take the action already long overdue.

Of course, all these human errors are costly. Americans spend billions of dollars a year on medical problems caused by outdoor pollution. And just as they decide to retreat inside their houses to find safety, there is the gas heater or fireplace, exuding harmful components inside buildings. There is no place like home -- and even more so the office -- for contaminated air. Many people suffer from "the sick-building syndrome." Pollution levels indoors, especially in buildings that have been "tightened" for energy conservation, are extremely high.

Toxic fumes enter the home or workplace in many ways. Newly installed carpets, furniture, plywood, and some foam insulation give off formaldehyde, causing headaches, impaired breathing, and irritated eyes and throat. Poorly vented kerosene heaters, gas ranges and wood stoves put out unhealthy amounts of carbon monoxide and nitrogen dioxide. Copying machines emit noxious ozone. Dry-cleaning fluids, disinfectants, paints and pesticides leak chemical vapors. Hazardous particles fill the air from cigarettes, dryers and abestos insulation. And we are not done yet. Fungi grow in cellars, bacteria may be drawn into air-conditioning systems from rooftop puddles or space above office ceilings.

The sources of damage are not easily removed. Legislation lags because fumes come from industries badly needed for the national economy and from automobiles and buses needed for private and public transportation. While we are thinking about tight budgets and profit-making industries, our Rome burns.

One of the most serious long-range environmental issues is the so-called **"Greenhouse effect."** Burning of forests and fossil fuels have increased the CO2 in the atmosphere. Scientists worry that the growing burden of CO2 and other gases may change the earth's climate. Like panes of glass in a greenhouse, CO2 allows more solar radiation to penetrate the atmosphere, but prevents part of the heat reflected by land and bodies of water from escaping into space. As CO2 accumulates, enough heat may be trapped to gradually warm the atmosphere. The rise of temperature could shift global rainfall patterns, bringing heavy rain to previously arid regions (Sahel in Africa) and droughts to productive farmlands such as the midwest. The impact could be even bigger at the poles where melting ice could gradually raise the ocean levels and flood many cities and farm regions.

We have mentioned Ozone as being damaging to our health. Yes, Ozone impairs vision and breathing when it occurs in smog. However, in the upper atmosphere, 30 miles above the ground, it protects life on earth by intercepting the sun's damaging ultraviolet radiation. Ozone is an unstable gas made of thre oxygen atoms stuck to gether. In past years, this protective layer of ozone has become thinner each spring over the Northern Hemisphere. Pictures taken from satellites show that a dark hole has been formed, within which ozone concentrations have fallen by 40 %. The potential effects can be serious: if the ozone continues to disappear, skin cancer incidence could rise sharply.

If a total loss of this ozone layer were to occur, we would have to take shelter under the sea or we would boil like lobsters. Not until this ozone layer was formed was life on land possible -- a frightening thought when we see how slow we are in altering our habits to avoid this catastrophe. The deadly mysterious hole of low-concentration ozone was barely discovered two years ago. It almost seems that the roof of the world has sprung a leak. Sunbathing could become a death-defying act, our immune system would falter, leaving us vulnerable to disease.

Furthermore, a radical loss of ozone might possibly render

the world uninhabitable. The stratosphere could heat up by as much as 40 degrees Farenheit, melting the polar ice caps. Sea levels would rise and submerge coastal cities. None of all this is a certainty, of course, but if things do not change, life on earth will never be the same.

Industrialists must have a self-destructive tendency, for the cause of depletion of the ozone layer is known: it is due to pollution from chemicals called Chlorofluorocarbons or CFCs. These are widely used in hairsprays, aerosol sprays, plastic foams, fire extinguishers, refrigeration systems and a host of other products which most of us consider essential to modern life.

How does it work? It is the "Pac-Man game" of our atmosphere. Each time a CFC molecule reaches the stratosphere, sunlight splits it into atoms of chlorine. The chlorine reacts with ozone to form oxygen and chlorine dioxyde (Cl+03...> 02 + Cl 02). The next insidious step is that chlorine oxide breaks up to form chlorine anew, which can again react with another ozone molecule (Cl 02...> Cl 2 + 02). A vicious Pac Man game, with one certain loser: human life.

September, 1987 saw a milestone in the annals of international politics. Forty nine nations met in Montreal, Canada. The result: an agreement to freeze, then eventually reduce their use of Chlorofluorocarbons, that destroy the ozone layer. That's the good news. The bad news is that even under the Montreal pact, which freezes CFC use at 1986 levels beginning in 1989 and cuts it 50% by 1999, the ozone layer will thin by about 2% in roughly seventy years, causing an estimated seven million extra cancer cases. Also, some loopholes in this treaty make it not as good as it looks. Developping countries will be allowed to increase CFC use 10% a year for ten years if that is vital to their economies. The only hope is that a search by manufacturers for substitutes may phase out the CFCs sooner than we can envision. It is my hope that the other environmental perils, the ocean pollution and the "greenhouse effect," previously discussed, will be tackled next.

Throughout history humans have lived with perils over which there seemed little control -- stronger creatures, hostile elements, mysterious diseases. One by one such threats have been tamed, increasing our confidence in our capabilities to survive hardships. This time the horrendous threat is of our own making. It is the modern "wolf at our door," and it might be the one that gets us.

2. POLLUTION OF OUR DRINKING WATER, RIVERS AND LAKES.

Water is our most needed nutrient, more important than vitamins and minerals or even food. It makes up more than half of our entire bodies (up to 65% in women, 75% in men, 85% in newborn infants). Not a cell in any of those bodies could function without it. It carries nourishing elements, including oxygen, into our bodies and gently removes wastes. Deprived of it, we could not live for a week.

Since this precious liquid is so vital a part of our very beings, we naturally treasure it, protect and preserve it, don't we? Not quite. Perverse creatures that we can sometimes be, we not only don't do those logical things, we misuse, abuse, waste and pollute our water. We even recklessly destroy its sources.

To begin with, we don't use this vital nutrient very wisely. We simply don't drink enough water. If you are average, your body contains between 40 and 50 quarts of water distributed over blood, muscles, brain and bones. You are constantly using up your internal reservoir, at an average rate of three quarts a day, through normal process of perspiration, excretion and sneezing, so you must constantly replenish it. A word of caution here. Don't depend on coffee or soft drinks for water replenishment. These are all diuretics, which cut your water ratio. The best choice would be fresh vegetable juices made on your own home juicer.

However, we are battling a little problem here. The EPA reports that three quarters of our own 180,000 waste disposal sites are leaking into underground water supplies. The Agency further estimates that 45% of large public water systems served by ground water are contaminated by organic chemicals. Half of our people depend on these systems. Each year, the toll of victims of water-borne diseases threatens to top 100,000. We still have the same amount of water we ever had on earth, plenty of it. The problem is that more of it has been made undrinkable -- by Nature and by Man.

Potential cancer-causing chemicals are also turning up in water supplies nationwide. Twenty-two chemicals so far have been identified by the EPA as cancer-causing. Luckily, only minute quantities have been discovered thus far. Of course, you do not need to wait on the government for action, which may be long in coming and longer in achieving any degree of effectiveness. You can protect your own household by (1) installing a filtration system; (2) building your own filtration system; or, (3) boiling all water for personal use.

Bottled water might be a solution, but it is not without faults. Remember that plastic is not an inert substance. Water sitting in plastic jugs can contain contaminants leached from the jug itself. Ideally, water should be stored in glass or stainless steel, and should be kept refrigerated. Some people feel safer with distilled water, but this is flat-tasting and contains no minerals, not even the beneficial ones. Reverse osmosis is another popular home-water treatment that comes with good and bad news. It removes essential minerals and trace minerals right along with asbestos and pesticide particles.

While we have problems with our drinking water, we seem to show even less respect for our rivers and lakes. Remember the toxic assault on the Rhine River in Germany on November 1, 1986. A fire destroyed the Sandoz Chemical Company warehouse in Basel, Switzerland, sending some 30 tons of pesticides, fungicides, herbicides and other toxic substances pouring into the Rhine River. Environmentalists were calling it the worst disaster in a decade. Over 300 kilometers of the Rhine were dead. A 60 kilometers slick of toxic chemicals had found its way downstream, poisoning a half million fish and 150.000 eels in its path. Most tragic was the fact that the Rhine was recovering from decades of near-sterility as a result of toxic pollution. A decade of effort was wiped out.

An investigation of the spill revealed some alarming facts: the Sandoz warehouse had no smoke or fire alarms, only two sprinklers and, most important, no adequate catch basins. The provisions for collecting run-off chemicals are "the single most crucial point" raised by the accident. When an insurance company advised corrective safety measures, Sandoz chose another carrier. The Sandoz disaster is only the most salient example of a toxic assault on the Rhine. The Rhine discharges some 100,000 tons of toxic chemicals and heavy metals into the North Sea each year.

U.S. environmental groups have similar stories. Sometimes, as was revealed by a "60 Minutes" investigation, the hazardous waste comes from a neighboring country, like Mexico. Of course, many of these polluting incidents go unnoticed or are never publicized. But even when they are, the stone walls of apathy remain our most formidable obstacle.

When we undertake to make our own households safe places to drink a glass of water, we will have made a beginning. When we concern ourselves with the state of water quality in our community, state, nation and world, we will have started a wholesome tide. We can never be complacent. Wherever in the world bad water exists, there lurks an enemy capable of launching horrible afflictions upon all of us.

3. EXPOSURE TO CIGARETTE SMOKE

"The most inflammatory question of our time," proclaimed the full page advertisements of a tobacco company last year. The question: "Hey, would you put out that cigarette?" To cigarette producers and to the nation's 60 million smokers, those sound like fighting words. But to nonsmokers, the request appears to be increasingly reasonable and justifiable.

At the beginning of 1987, in the Public Health Servive's annual report on smoking, U.S. Surgeon-General C. Everett Koop warned that so-called "involuntary" smoking -- simply breathing in the vicinity of people with lighted cigarettes in enclosed areas -- can cause lung cancer and other illnesses to healthy nonsmokers. Children of parents who smoke, the report stated, have more respiratory infections than children of nonsmokers. Infants of parents who smoke are hospitalized more often for pneumonia and bronchitis than babies in nonsmoking households. Furthermore, the risk of involuntary smoke inhalation may not be eliminated by separating nonsmokers from smokers within the same air space, a revelation that will certainly come as no surprise to frequent nonsmoking air passengers or restaurant patrons who are seated near smoking sections.

It is now clear that disease risk due to inhalation of tobacco smoke is not solely limited to the individual who is smoking. It should be obvious to all that the right of the smoker to smoke stops at the point where his or her smoking increases the disease risk of those occupying the immediate area. The National Academy of Sciences suggests that this factor may be responsible for 2400 lung cancer deaths annually. I call these deaths simply aggravated assault, even murder. These and other data, derived from dozens of studies that have appeared in scientific literature over the past several years, should fuel the campaign by doctors and antismoking advocates to impose more restrictions on smoking in the workplace and in public buildings and conveyances.

Of course, this type of report draws the criticism of cigarette manufacturers, who call these data "inconclusive and incomplete." The manufacturers are the same people who objected to the landmark 1964 report of the Surgeon General, linking smoking to lung cancer, of which there is now strong evidence. How long do we have to wait for action?

4. MEDICATIONS

In the USA, it has been calculated that more people are killed each year by prescribed drugs than by accidents on the roads. "Iatrogenic" or "Doctor-caused" disease is an enormous and growing medical problem. When it appears, the doctor's usual response, alas, is yet another medication, with its own side effects. The traditional role of the physician has been distorted by the ready availability of drugs. Every patient walking into the office of his doctor expects the doctor to get out the prescription pad. Generally, it is the easy way out for doctor and patient. The patient wants to forget that a lot of work has to be done in order to reach maximum health. He demands from his doctor a magic pill, a cure-all that will take away all the suffering instantly. And many doctors believe that reliance on drugs is the answer.

Let's face it. Drugs are manufactured by commercial organizations for the same reason as any other product: to make a profit. Drug companies make money, billions of dollars, by selling drugs. Primarly, they are not interested in your health, which in the USA is reflected in the attitudes of insurance companies: the cost of preventive medicine and supplements is not covered. Preventive medicine is the only true form of medicine, but apart from vaccinations, little attention is paid to this aspect of medical science.

Much attention has been paid to the increased use of marijuna, LSD, crack, heroin and cocaine. Considering the number of crimes related to these drugs, our society seems to be taking a turn for the worse. Yet whatever one may feel about the abuse of illegal drugs, it is not the real problem. Today's drug addict can be the nice neighbor, the person next to you on the bus, the co-worker you like so much. It can even be you who may come to depend on drugs. One of the places where you can become addicted to medications, especially sleeping pills and relaxants, is the place where you go to restore your health: the hospital. Thousands of people are introduced for the first time to Valium, Librium or Halcion and are hooked on the for the rest of their lives. A big price to be paid for trying to get well! The change has to come from the patient: there has to be an increased awareness of the toxic side effects of drugs. Question your doctor, read about the drug and ask for an alternative if you don't like what you hear or read.

When Paul Ehrlich, a German phycisian, used Salvarsan as the first available drug to fight syphillis, initially he called it a "magic bullet." He visualized that he was firing a bullet into the invading enemy, without doing harm to the healthy cells. It is ironic that while Ehrlich almost immediatly abandoned the idea, modern doctors still adhere to this simplistic solution. Ehrlich stated: "it is highly likely that artificially-produced substances, foreign to the body, will be attracted also by the organs, and these substances are not unlikely to injure the organism as a whole." I am convinced that many patients would refuse to take certain medications if they were informed by their doctors about the possible side-effects.

While side-effects relating to symptoms such as dry mouth,

impotence, nausea, vomiting, diarrhea, impaired hair growth, (the list is endless) are bad enough, we really are getting into trouble when we look at the medications affecting our immune system. It is incredible that for diseases such as cancer -- an expression of our depleted immune system -- medications are prescribed that suppress the bone marrow, decreasing the amount of white blood cells, our first line defenders of the immune system.

One thing that makes the doctor more confident when he prescribes drugs is the thought that he has an antidote available. What a misconception! Only rarely do we have an antidote available, and treatment is therefore based on symptomatic, supportive measures. Tissue damage frequently occurs, unfortunatly often irreversible. It took a long time for the medical profession to accept that for barbiturate (sleeping pills) intoxication, prescribing stimulants was not the right answer. A study done in a specialized centrum in Denmark in 1960 discovered that death rates doubled when stimulants were given.

Discussing all the side-effects of medications goes beyond the scope of this book. Rather, I will concentrate on the more commonly used drugs, those affecting our immune system and triggering diseases such as EBV, Candida, Herpes simplex and other immune-suppressed-related conditions.

ANTIBIOTICS

Antibiotics are chemicals that interfere with the life processes of pathogenic microorganisms, prevent their multiplication by interrupting their reproduction, and occasionally destroy the pathogens. The treatment of infections with what we would now call antibiotics has been known for thousands of years. Ancient Chinese savants treated boils, carbuncles and other skin infections with moldy soybean decoctions, the mold serving as a source of antibiotic.

The best-known antibiotic, and the first of its kind, was discovered by British bacteriologist Alexander Fleming in September, 1928. A culture of staphylococci growing on an agar medium became contaminated by a mold that had been carried to it in the laboratory air from some distance. The bacteria growing in the vicinity of the mold disappeared. Fleming identified the mold as Penicillium Notatum and realized it must have produced an antibiotic substance, which he named penicillin. This discovery was the onset of the now widespread use and abuse of antibiotics. In spite of all the good results they have brought, adverse reactions have become common place. There are probably 30,000 deaths per year due to adverse reactions to antibiotics in U.S. hospitals alone. The hazards of antibiotics use are not restricted to the individual patient. Environmental pollution due to the unrestrained use of antibiotics results in the development of antibiotic-resistant strains of bacteria. These are bred in centers of high antibiotic use as divergent as pig farms and the surgical wards of major hospitals.

One of the greatest problems that antibiotic use has created is the present epidemic of Candida Albicans and Tropicalis. Candida Albicans is a yeast-like fungus whose habitat is the mucosae of warm-blooded animals and humans. In individuals whose immune system are intact the organism is typically benign. The frightening thing about Candida is that it can detect weaknesses in our immune system a lot faster than we can with our chemical tests. The previous sentence speaks volumes about the tendency of Candida Albicans to become extremely opportunistic. Prolonged broad spectrum antibacterial therapy, using tetracyclines in particular, results in a replacement of the natural flora of friendly bacteria. Instead, resistant organisms, including yeasts, will be predominant. (For more about Candida Albicans, see Chapter three)

Tetracycline is one of the most commonly prescribed drugs in this country. It is handed out almost like candy. One of its major indications is that it is prescribed in chronic low doses for acne. Many victims now between the ages of 30 and 40 are suffering the horrible consequences: a chronic yeast condition, leading eventually to a totally-weakened immune system. Now, it does not bother me if an adult is stupid enough to be hoodwinked by slick advertising into taking some worthless cold remedy. But it really raises my ire when well-meaning parents encourage trusting adolescents to swallow a potentially-hazardous concoction.

Of course, not all the criticism should be leveled at parents. On the contrary, the biggest part of the blame lies with the drug companies that seem to care more about the health of their profits than the well-being of their customers. Also some of the blame belongs to doctors who, through ignorance, stupidity or convenience, prescribe damaging drugs for children. The classical example of physician incompetence is the continued prescribing of tetracyclines for relatively minor illnesses such as bronchitis or sore throats. Doctors have known for more than twenty years that this broad-spectrum antibiotic has serious and long-lasting side-effects. There are few, if any, reasons for prescribing this drug to children under 8 years old. It causes permanent discoloration of the teeth (yellow-brown).

In spite of this, studies have shown that prescribing of tetracyclines for children under age 8, remains widespread! This is not just shocking, it is downright criminal. It is hard to understand why the FDA allows drug companies to fabricate tetracycline syrups aimed at this age group. And don't tell me it is because older people often require the liquid form. Studies and statistics show that 60% of these prescriptions are for children, under 9 years old.

Parents, be aware of the fact that tetracyclines are available in many different brand-name preparations. It is virtually impossible for parents to know whether they are giving their child this type of antibiotic unless a physician tells them so. Don't be afraid to ask your doctor: you owe it to your child. Aureomycin, Terramycin, Vibramycin, Tetrex, Tetracyn and Semocyclin are just a few of these brand names. Please, parents, do not think that I am making a mountain out of a molehill on this tetracycline issue. Far from it. Besides the distraught children who have to live a lifetime with ugly teeth, millions are now affected by systematic yeast infections because of tetracycline used in their childhood.

Another immune damaging class of antibiotics is the sulphonamides. Brand names are Septrin and Bactrim. These are prescribed particularly for chronic bronchitis and urinary tract infections. Both these conditions require long-term medication, which is unfortunate in view of the fact that adverse reactions to these kinds of medications are more likely to occur with prolonged use. Sulphonamides can cause blood disorders resulting from damage to blood cells, pigment and blood marrow, the production place of our immune system defenders.

One of the surest place in this world to get infections is in the hospital. Germs that never would attack you on the outside, because they are less frequently present, lurk in every corner of the hospital, endangering all patients, especially the elderly. To fight these Klebsiella, Proteus, Pseudomonas and other potent germs with esoteric names, often mixtures of antibiotics and drugs harmful to the immune system are prescribed. A few of these are Gentamicin, Keflin and Chloramphenicol. All these medications can cause a bone marrow depression, leading to neutropenia (a lack of white blood cells), thrombocytopenia (a lack of platelets) and aplastic anemia with a lack of all the blood-forming elements. There have been reports of aplastic anemia later developing into leukemia.

CORTISONE

We are aware of the enormous potential of this drug in life-threatening situations, such as poisoning, allergic shock, asthma crisis, etc... However, the dangers of cortisone loom over the patient, almost entirely cancelling its advantages. Systematic corticosteroid therapy causes Cushing's disease, diabetes, stomach ulcers and bleeding, masks infections, delays wound healing and above all (important for us here), causes a fluctuation in the peripheral lymphocytes (defender white blood cells), which exerts an immunosuppressive effect that increases the risk of Candidiasis.

And if you only think about the tablet and injection form of cortisone, then you should know that the much used -- and over-the-counter-available -- cortisone skin cream produces the same effect. On the skin itself, continued use of these creams produces peeling of deep layers, creating a depressed, striped area. It often leads to an irreversible atrophy of the skin. Another side effect on the skin is the formation of cortisone-acne. Cortisone seems marvellously effective, but its long-term use entails hazards both through local effects at the site of application and through absorption into the general circulation.

INDOMETHACIN (INDOCID)

I do not know of a bigger money-making item for the pharmaceutical industry than the arthritis-related drugs. Income from these medications runs into billions of dollars. Now that some of them are available over-the-counter, the danger of overdosing seems imminent.

People tend to think that these drugs are merely a fortified aspirin, to be taken at the slightest discomfort. However, one of the greatest dangers is the incidence of aplastic anemia: a decrease of all the blood-forming elements, often with fatal consequences. Indomethacin is also believed to be capable of masking infection and activating latent infection. So each time you take one of those pills, think about a possible time bomb you may be putting into your immune system. Because of deaths from infections arising in the course of diseases (such as arthritis, rheumatic fever, etc...), indomethacin should be banned for children.

ANTI-CANCER DRUGS

Cancer is not one disease but an estimated group of over one hundred diseases affecting different organs. For such a variety of diseases there must be a variety of causes: environmental, dietary, hereditary and emotional factors. All these factors lead to one result: a permanent change in a cell that causes errors in the direction of constructing genes or making proteins. Unfortunatly, after many years and billions of dollars' worth of research, our main attack on these cancer cells consists of radiation, surgery and chemotherapy. It is the latter option that we must take a closer look at.

Chemotherapy can induce prolonged remissions of cures in a substantial proportion of patients with Hodgkin's disease, leukemia of childhood, and Burkitt's lymphoma. Lesser improvements are achieved in other neoplasms as well. But at what price?

Leukeran, Cytoxan, Alkeran, Myleran, Methotrexate, Purinethol, 5-Fluorouracil, and Velban are the major medications used in the treatment of various cancers. All of them have a bone-marrow-suppressing effect; in other words, they cause a decrease in the number of white blood cells, red blood cells and platelets. The most fearsome effect is again the decreased number of white blood cells. This weakening of the immune system in already weakened patients throws the door wide open to viruses, bacteria and yeast cells. It is no surprise, therefore, that many of these unfortunate people succumb to secondary infections.

Is there an alternative? I think that besides the use of these often effective medications, all the other aspects (especially the emotional) of disease as outlined before should be taken in consideration. I strongly believe that if we want to get control of this giant killer that causes 600,000 deaths a year in the USA (talk about an epidemic!), we must improve our food quality, our soil, our environments and our emotions. In other words, without a drastic change in life-style, we will not prevail.

5. LIFE - STYLE CHANGES

Life-style is one factor the Chinese did not include in their system of medicine 5000 years ago. But it is my strong belief that the extraordinary life-style change in the 60's was one of the main triggering factors in the incidence of the present immuno-suppressed diseases. It makes sense when we see that the majority of the victims of CEBV, CMV, Candida and Herpes Simplex viruses are between 30 and 45 years old.

The 60's brought drugs into the mainstream, promoting the use of marijuana in the first place. This quickly led to the intake of other abused substances such as cocaine and heroin. All these drugs create "Heat-Dampness" in the body, disrupting the natural balance of the internal organs, especially the liver and the spleen-pancreas.

The 60's also was a time of "sexual liberation" leading to easier and more promiscuous sexual encounters, increasing sexually-transmitted deseases such as gonorrhea, syphilis and especially Herpes Simplex 2 or genital herpes. All these infections. either because of the intake of antibiotics or because of the latent presence of the virus, decreased the strength of the immune system, making its victims more susceptible to the recent surge of EBV and Candida. In fact, most patients today have viruses and yeast cells present at the same time.

D. EMOTIONS

1. IMMUNE DISEASES AND THE MIND

More than in any other form of medicine, acupuncture looks at the psyche of the patient, knowing and recognizing its importance to restore health. In fact, as far as the Chinese are concerned, any disease starts with a psychological disturbance.

Thus while we still struggle in Western medicine to unlock the secrets of emotions in the pathogenesis of disease, 5000 years ago the Chinese discovered the close relationship between emotions and the healthy functioning of the different organs. For the Chinese, there are seven emotional factors:

ANGER

JOY

PENSIVENESS

GRIEF

MELANCHOLY

WORRY

FEAR

When these emotions are in balance, there is no psychological disorder. In fact, even a healthy individual needs to express each of these emotions to a certain degree: only then is s/he emotionally well-balanced. Who needs fear, you ask. If we did not have fear, we would not survive long. A healthy amount of fear is what keeps us on our toes when we encounter dangerous situations. On the other hand, too much fear would immobilize us, leaving us helpless and without the ability to react. Hence, the importance of finding a balance in our emotions.

The Chinese knew that each emotion was linked to a certain organ. This relationship has radical consequences. Too much of a particular emotion will damage the correlated organ. Moreover, once that emotion decreases the energy in the corresponding organ, the weakness in this organ will lead to an increase of the emotion itself. Let me give you an example. Fear leads to a decrease of energy in the kidney. When the kidney becomes weaker, patients with this condition will experience even more fear, completing the vicious circle. The physical disturbances which this can lead to will be fully outlined in "Autoimmune diseases and the mind."

These are the relationships between the seven basic emotions and their corresponding organs:

Too much anger will injure the liver.

Too much joy will injure the heart.

Too much grief and melancholy will injure the lung.

Too much fear will injure the kidney.

Too much pensiveness and worry will injure the spleen-pancreas.

Thus the most important emotions for the immune system are pensiveness and worry, which are linked to the spleen-pancreas. Too much worry leads to a suppressed immune sytem, thus leading us into catastrophic diseases. This means that the type-A obsessive and compulsive personality is a potential candidate for immune-suppressed diseases. People with type-A personalities are excessively competitive and seem to have a continual sense of time urgency, accompanied by the feeling of always having to meet deadlines. As a result, they have no patience with people who delay them by taking too much time to do a job. Type-A individuals will show an easily-aroused hostility, usually well rationalized and for the most part under control. Type-A individuals are aggressive and extroverted, dominating gatherings and conversations. Do you recognize yourself? If so, you are well on your way to suppressing your immune system!

I firmly believe that Western medical practitioners will get nowhere in combatting cancer, AIDS, EBV, etc... , if we do not take into account the emotional factors affecting the immune system. Our tendency is to explain everything on a physiological basis, which is an insult to the human being: the mind is much more powerful than the body.

Western civilisations tend to emphasize the individual parts of man rather than seeing him as an integrated whole. When we look at the present structure of our healing professions, we see that things have gotten out of hand. At first, we had two large groups: physicians, dedicated to the treatment of the body, while psychiatrists and psychologists concentrated on healing the mind. Now, however, we have sub-specialities in specialities, such as neuro-ophtalmologists – doctors only concerned with neurological disorders of the eyes. The misconception here is to regard mind and body as totally distinct entities. Five thousand years ago, the Chinese approached the individual as a physically, psychologically, and spiritually integrated being while gaining as much understanding as possible about his relationship with his environment. Fortunatly, a new breed of doctor is appearing in Western medicine: the holistic doctor, who like the ancient Chinese treats the person as an integrated unit and studies his psycho-social environment. These doctors still rely on modern diagnostic tests, but their approach is also humanistic and emphasizes the patient rather than technology.

The equivalent of **worry** in Chinese medicine is **stress** in Western medicine. It is the rate of "wear and tear" within the body, present in any living organism. Blame whatever you will -- jobs, spouses, bills, kids, the complexity of life -- stress has become one of America's most common health problems. Pressure, pressure everywhere! Especially in our "yuppie" society, psycho-social stress has become a dangerously cumulative phenomenon. Many of the major precursors of stress are readily apparent: death of a spouse or other family member, divorce, separation, personal injury. Others, not viewed as stress factors but as positive and even pleasurable events, can be just as stress-inducing as those considered negative: marriage, retirement, vacation, pregnancy, or a new addition to the family.

People's attitudes about illnesses and life itself have biochemical effects. For the same effort, we either choose to have the healing powers of laughter and emotional well-being or the destructive effects of panic and depression. Not only human beings, but also every other living creature is exposed to stress. Physiologically, we have the same defense mechanisms against stress as animals: either we accept the challenge of the stress and we fight it, or we decide not to be exposed to it and run away from it.

Theoretically, this fight-or-flight model is the same in all living creatures. Practically, however, human beings have to deal with stress by fighting or accepting it. Flight from imminent stress is socially unacceptable. When you have an argument with your wife, and you feel that you would like to get rid of her, you cannot assault her or just walk away without consequences. Stress on your job has to be suppressed because of fear of losing the job. So in spite of an outward calm, your body is entering a state of anger and rage because you may not have a socially-acceptable action to take.

How does this affect your immune system? When the sympathetic nervous system is activated in response to stress, it works in close relationship with the endocrine system, and particularly with the hypotalamus, located in the brain. Stress will release a stimulating factor from the hypotalamus which will act on the pituitary gland, located at the base of the brain. This gland secretes hormones into the bloodstream which carry specific messages to other endocrine glands. One of those factors is ACTH or the adreno-corticotrophic factor, acting on the adrenal cortex. One of the factors that increases in response to ACTH is cortisone. We have already mentioned the negative effects of cortisone (Page # 51). We know that the prolonged presence of cortisone will seriously interfere with the effectiveness of the immune system. This biofeedback mechanism of the endocrine system is shown in Fig. # 5.

Most likely, stress affects mainly the macrophages, our major

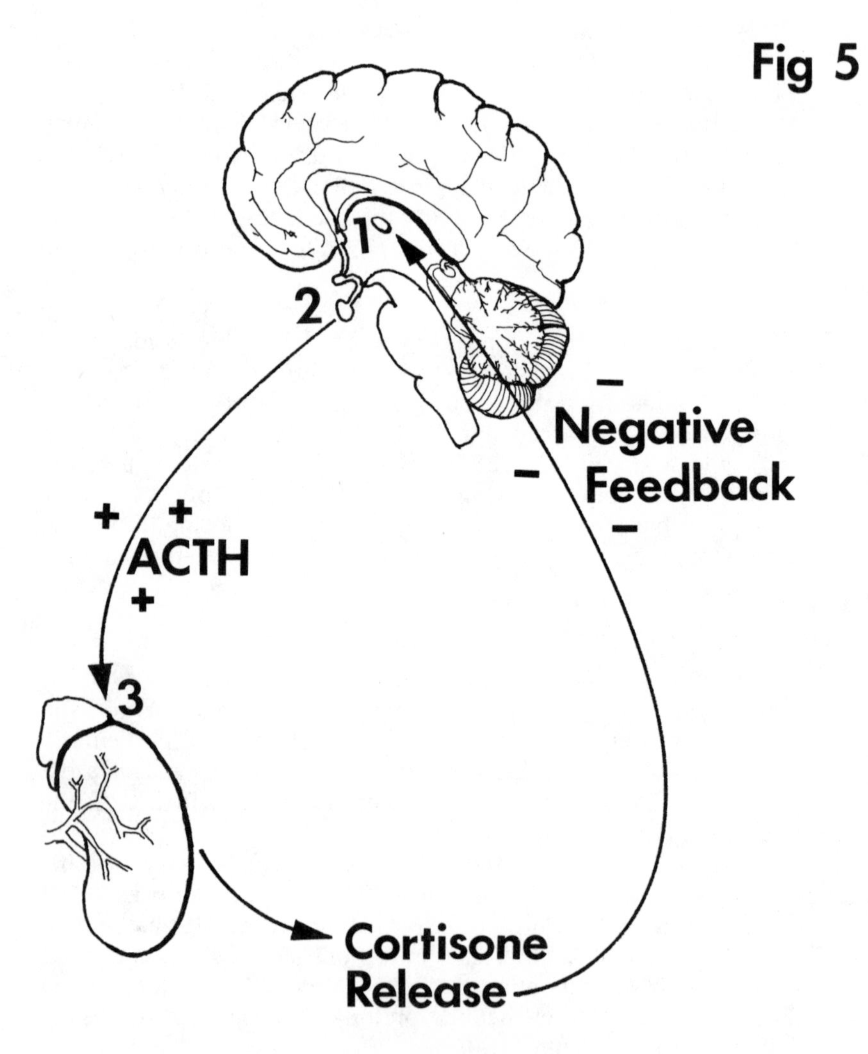

1. Hypothalamus
2. Pituitary Gland
3. Adrenal Cortex

clean-up police force. Other results observed in lab animals includes an enlargement of the adrenal cortex, a shrinkage of the thymus and changes in the spleen and lymph nodes: all omnipresent signs of damage to the body when under attack. These relatively small changes in the immunological balance can shift the entire system and predispose an individual to the development of disease. And we know that yeast cells and viruses detect these subtle changes a lot faster than our lab tests, giving them an edge on our defense system.

Now that there is a lot of medical evidence establishing the negative effect of emotions -- depression, anger, panic, hate, exasperation -- we have to start realizing that hope, the will to live, creativity and laughter -- in short, people's attitude toward illness and life itself -- will have positive biochemical effects. In Houston, Texas, a world-famous cancer center, children play video-games in which they can see on a screen how their helper T-cells attack cancer cells. With a scoring system, they can visualize how they can fight back. It takes away the feeling of helplessness those children might experience, giving them instead a sense that they are actively participating in the battle with cancer.

2. AUTOIMMUNE DISEASES AND THE MIND

If the immune system does not give us enough secrets to unlock, there is a group of diseases that is even more mind-boggling and mysterious: the autoimmune diseases. What triggers these illnesses is that there are enough Helper T-cells but not enough Suppressor T-cells (T8) to call the battle off. In fact, the battle should not be a battle: the body starts recognizing its own tissues as antigens or strange objects and forms antibodies against its own cell structures. The list of autoimmune diseases is long and certainly incomplete at this time. In the future, when the immune system reveals more of its secrets, many more pathologies will fill this mysterious list. We have already R.A. (Rheumatoid Arthritis), SLE (Systematic Lupus Erythomatosis), Scleroderma, M.S. (Multiple Sclerosis), Hashimoto's disease (a thyroid disfunction), Crohn's disease, Colitis Ulcerosa, Bechterew disease, Periarteritis nodosa, Morbus Reiter and Glomerulonephritis (a kidney disease).

The one group that has been studied the most extensively, most likely because of the great numbers of people involved, is the rheumatoid Arthritis group. These studies have identified that patients are belonging to a certain bio-type. Studying the cases in my practice and recalling the attitude of acupuncture toward these patients 5000 years ago, I was interested in the events that took place just prior to the outbreak of a first rheumatic attack. My question to my patients was: "What happened a couple of months prior to your first attack -- was there a major psychological trauma in your life?" From my study of acupuncture medicine, I was sure there would be one. The emotions linked to the kidney organ (which is the organ linked to the bones in acupuncture), are fear and anxiety. In other words, any trauma triggering these emotions with enough intensity sets the patient up for this disastrous condition. We have already alluded to the different triggering factors. In order of severity they are:

Death of a spouse

Divorce

Marital separation

Death of a close family member

The Chinese identified "kidney deficient" or arthritis-prone people as indecisive in nature, extremely dependent, possessing feelings of inadequacy and severely blocked in their emotional expressions.

Unfortunatly, rheumatic disease hits our children as well. In one survey it was seen that in children who had a traumatic childhood (death, separation or divorce of the parents), the incidence of RA was a lot higher. Thus it can be related to the fear and anxiety such children go through as they feel abandoned. For children tend to blame themselves in case of divorce or death, feeling that if it was not for them, these separations would not have taken place.

Considering these triggering factors and the relationship between the condition and traumatic emotions, it is no wonder that we have made no "big advances" in treating arthritis with medication. These "magic bullets" simply are too narrowly focussed on physiological symptoms. On the other hand, acupuncture treatments have proven very effective, simply because besides treating the root of the problem -- the weakness in the kidney organ -- the acupuncturist will also recocgnize the need of appropriate nutrition, psychotherapy and exercise.

3. THE BODY-MIND CONNECTION`

The seventeenth-century French philosopher Rene Descartes strongly influenced the course of modern medicine. One of his perceptions was that body and mind were two separate entities, not unitary and interlocked. Even famous immunologists still adhere to this principle: they picture the immune system operating outside the control of the brain or central nervous system. In this perspective, the patient's success in fighting off disease will depend on the strength of his body defenses, not his mind's.

Yet for centuries anecdotal evidence has accumulated to indicate that the mind can indeed influence a person's vulnerability to disease. The Chinese, as we have noted, were even able to connect specific emotions with specific organs (page # 55). We don't have to go back that far to see a documented relationship between body and mind. The "placebo" effect has had a long-time recognized place in medical practice, and stories in which doctors achieve miraculous cures with placebos have been repeatedly documented. (The "placebo" is a technique often use in medicine to wean people away from addictive medications by supplying them with a "sugar" pill that has no pharmaceutically-known action or effect). Today, inspite of some lingering skepticism, more and more evidence points to the existence of intimate ties between the central nervous system and the immune system. This new discipline of medicine is frequently called "Psychoneuroimmunology." It does not really make sense to think that two systems so exquisitely designed to protect our organism would not also be related.

Many experiments have been (and are being) conducted merely to show the key role that the central nervous system plays in the regulation and control of the immune system. Robert Ader, of the university of Rochester School of Medicine and Dentistry, for instance, studied the effect of psycho-social factors in early life on subsequent vulnerability to disease **(Ref. # 1).** Ader let rats drink saccharin solution, immediatly followed by an injection of cyclophosphamide (Cytoxan), wich induces nausea-like disturbances. (Cytoxan is a medication used in cancer therapy, specifically in the treatment of Hodgkin's for example). After just one such experience, rats would choose plain water over the saccharin water, since they associated the taste of saccharin with getting sick. This should not come as surprise, because the survival of animals in the wild depends on their ability to recognize these toxic factors in their environment.

In the next step, Ader continued to give the saccharin water without Cytoxan and observed that it gradually weakened their conditioning -- nothing unusual. What was unexpected, however, was that several weeks into the study those rats that continued to drink the flavored solution became sick. It is known that Cytoxan suppresses immune functions, but it seemed strange that these animals' immune systems were weakened weeks after they received the one and only dose of cyclophosphamide.

Ader then used various control groups. Some rats received plain water with their cyclophosphamide, and only later the saccharin; some got the saccharin and cyclophosphamide together, but so widely apart that they could not learn to associate one with the other. None of the above groups suffered as much damage to the immune system as did the conditioned group. Other immunologists balked at this results and stated that the immune-suppressed effects were too small to be statistically significant. However, Ader could reproduce these effects over and over again. Perhaps small differences are not what immunologists are dealing with, but at this point, with the vast array of immuno-suppressed diseases, even a 10% change becomes important.

But in nature, this is not how things work out: you do not get invariably ill when you are exposed to pathogens. There are other factors involved as discussed before: hereditary factors, emotions, social influences, exterior factors and food intake.

These factors, presumably through the nervous system, modulate the immune system. One well-established mechanism, the hypotalamus-pituitary-adrenal cortex axis, is explained on page # 57. But researchers were not pleased with the above pathway only; they felt there ought to be direct pathways between the central nervous system and the immune sysytem. In experiments the thymus of a rat was injected with horseradish peroxidase. Under the microscope, this horseradish could be traced directly to several groups of neurons in the brain stem and the spinal cord, hinting at links between the nervous and immune systems.

Another study was done at Mt. Sinai School of Medicine in New York City by Drs. Stein, Schleifer and Keller. After conducting successful animal tests, they picked the death of spouse, the number one stress factor for human beings (page # 60) to see how stress would influence the strength of the immune system. Their subjects were all husbands of women with advanced breast cancer. Following the death of the men's wives, a weakening of immune response was noted, returning to normal over the course of the following year. In the past these subtle changes might not have meant too much to some researchers. However, in the light of the killer immuno-deficiency disease, AIDS, more and more people will respect these changes in the strength of the immune sysytem, however modest.

For some scientists, neuroimmunoligy is still a field of "witchcraft" and for "quacks." However, it is my opinion that scientific "tunnel vision," and the penchant for dividing the body into compartments, will delay solutions for millions of people suffering from immunosuppressed diseases. Western medicine will do well to add "peripheral vision" to its "tunnel vision" in order to illuminate ties involved in neuro-immunomodulation.

Ref # 1: "Behaviorally Conditioned Immunosuppression and Murine Lupus Erythomatosus", Robert Ader, M.D. and Nicholas Cohen, M.D.; Department of Microbiology, University of Rochester School of Medicine and Dentistry, 1982.

3. HOW TO DETERMINE THE STRENGTH OF OUR IMMUNE SYSTEM

"How strong is my immune system?" is probably the most frequently asked question nowadays. In this chapter I will explain what laboratory tests can tell us, and also, how a self-scoring questionnaire can give us some insight into the strength of the mind/ body's defense mechanism.

A. LABORATORY TESTS

Aside from special blood tests in cases of Candida, EBV, CMV, and Herpes Simplex 1 and 2 (which are discussed further in chapters 3 and 4), the physician can ask for a **"Complete Immune Panel."** I will explain step-by-step how to interpret these findings. The immune panel consists of the total white blood cell (WBC) count, the total lymphocytes, the T4 or Helper T-cells, the T8 or Suppressor T-cells, the T4/T8 ratio and the total B-lymphocytes.

WBC count:

This is simply a count of the number of white blood cells in a given amount of blood. As explained in (A), these white blood cells form the bulk of your defenders. They are the "cell-eaters": macrophages and neutrophils, the "killer" cells and the antibody-forming structures. Depending on the reference rates of the lab, a normal number is between 4,000 and 11,000 WBC/cu mm. In other words, when you go below 4,000, it indicates a weakness in your immune system: you simply have too few soldiers to throw into the battle. On the other hand, an increase in WBC (more than 11,000) is a sign of infection, with an adequate response of your immune system.

Total Lymphocytes:

These are the T-and B-cells, the cornerstones of your immune system. They are normally a certain percentage (25-40%) of your WBC. Again, a decrease in this percentage indicates a weakened immune system.

T4 or Helper T-cells:

They are the generals of our immune system, calling upon the other cells (B-cells, Killer T-cells) to help fight the enemy. Normally they are between 35-55% of the Lymphocytes. If your figure is far below the 35%, it means that your immune system is compromised; not enough Helper T-cells will call for help, hence the attacker (virus, yeast cell, bacteria), has more time to multilply and further weaken your resistance. An extreme example will be AIDS, where most of the Helper T-cells are knocked out since the AIDS virus has been able to slip into this cell. As a result, the Helper T-cells are not giving any messages to the rest of the troops. On the other hand, a figure above 55% indicates an "overreactive" or "hyperreactive" immune system, where too many Helper T-cells are summoned to fight a troup of enemies. If this continues, the number of Helper T-cells will become exhausted, leading to the exhaustion of the immune system.

Suppressor T-cells or T8 cells:

These soldiers have to call the fight off when the battle is won; their normal figure is between 20 and 37% of the Lymphocytes; too few T8 cells will cause the battle to continue unnecessarily, again exhausting the number of T4 cells.

T4 / T8 Ratio:

Ideally, you want 1.8 T4 cells for every one T8 cell; in other words, the ratio will be roughly 1.8/1 or simply 1.8. If the ratio falls, you don't have enough T4 cells prodding the immune system into action.

B-Cells:

These are the "factories" where the antibodies are formed that slow down or neutralize the invaders. The normal amount is 5-25% of the total Lymphocytes. Absence of B-cells or markedly reduced numbers are suggestive of immunodeficiency states. A marked increase is suggestive of malignancy states and helpful in the diagnosis of Chronic Lynphocytic Leukemia (CLL).

Interleukin-2:

This is a glycoprotein released by the Helper T-cells. Functions of Interleukin-2 include T-cell proliferation, stimulation of interferon and B-cell growth factor, all very important in our defenses system. The inability of the human T-cell to generate normal amounts of IL-2 is diagnostic of immunodeficiency seen in conditions such as AIDS, Candida, SLE (Systematic Lupus Erythomatosis), Pemphigus and T-cell Leukemias.

The above findings are expressed in table # 4.

Table # 4

Cell Type	N1	Decreased	Increased
WBC	4,000-11,000	Too few defenders	Sign of infection
Lympho's	25-40% of WBC	Immune system down	Infection or cancer
T4	35-55% of Lympho's	The general of the immune system forgets to alert his troops	Overreactive immune system
T8	20-37% of Lympho's	Battles continues	Battle called off too early
T4/T8 Ratio	1.8	Suppressed immunity	Too many T4 or too few T8 cells
B-cells	5-25% of Lympho's	Not enough enemies neutralized	Overreactive immune system or cancer
Interleukin-2		Suppressed immunity	

B. A SELF SCORING QUESTIONNAIRE

The following is a self-scoring test that consists of two parts: first, the triggering factors leading to a weakened immune system, and secondly, the different symptoms and signs of a weakened defense system.

Completing this questionnaire will be a good indicator of where you stand in respect to your immune system. Read the questionnaire and add up the score based on how the answers apply to your own life story.

If you score between 0 and 150, congratulations! You have been taking care of your immune system, most likely through an excellent life-style. It is very unlikely that you have any of the immunosuppressed conditions present.

If your score is between 150 and 300, you are moving towards calamity -- too many triggering factors most probably have already weakened your immune system. It is high time to make life-style changes, because you might be already suffering from one or more immunosuppressed conditions.

If your score is between 300 and 600, there is a very great chance that you suffer from one or more immunosuppressed conditions. Consult your doctor immediatly and ask for the appropriate tests (see page 64 and page ... of chapter six). Life-style changes are imperative!

If your score is between 600 and 1,200, filling out this questionnaire brought you no news; you know you are not doing well, to say the least. What you might not have known is that you are suffering from an immunosuppressed condition. Seeking help from your physician is critical.

A. TRIGGERING FACTORS

a. Hereditary factors

Have one of your parents or sibblings suffered from one of the following diseases? (10 points on each "yes")

✧ Manic-depressive disorder

✧ Diabetes mellitus

✧ Rheumatoid Arthritis

✧ Low thyroid function

✧ Cancer in any form

✧ Hypoglycemia

✧ Allergies

✧ Lupus Erythematosis

✧ Scleroderma

✧ Hashimoto's disease

✧ Pemphigus vulgaris

✧ Idiopathic Thrombocytopenic Purpura

b. Emotional factors

PERSONALITY (5 points on each "yes")

✧ Are you competitive?

✧ Are you impatient and driven?

✧ Is your hostility easily aroused?

- ✧ Are you obsessive about exercise?
- ✧ Are you nervous and easily frustrated?
- ✧ Do you judge accomplishments in numbers?
- ✧ Do you have difficulty taking time for genuine leisure?
- ✧ Are you aggressive?
- ✧ Are you extroverted?
- ✧ Do you dominate conversations?
- ✧ Are you insecure about yourself?
- ✧ Do you hate to be disliked?
- ✧ Are you hardworking?
- ✧ Are you overly analytical?
- ✧ Are you obsessed with the past?

STRESS-TRIGGERING FACTORS

Have you recently (in the last year) experienced:

- ✧ Death of spouse (25 points)
- ✧ Divorce (20 points)
- ✧ Death of a close family member (15 points)
- ✧ Marital separation (15 points)
- ✧ Jail term (15 points)
- ✧ Personal injury (12 points)
- ✧ Marriage (12 points)

- ✧ Dismissal from your job (12 points)
- ✧ Retirement (10 points)
- ✧ Pregnancy (10 points)
- ✧ Sex difficulties (10 points)
- ✧ Mortgage or loan over $100,000 (8 points)
- ✧ Trouble with in-laws (8 points)
- ✧ Trouble with boss (5 points)
- ✧ Change in residence, working hours, habits or activities (5 points)
- ✧ Were you in the past the victim of child-abuse? (15 points)
- ✧ Were one or both of your parents alcoholics?

c. Nutritional factors

- ✧ Are you addicted to sugar, Nutrasweet, or chocolate? (20 points)
- ✧ Do you have cravings for bread? (10 points)
- ✧ Do you omit breakfast? (10 points)
- ✧ Do you eat products containing white flour? (10 points)
- ✧ Do you have irregular eating habits? (10 points)
- ✧ Do you eat a lot of fried foods? (10 points)
- ✧ Do you rarely eat fresh fruits? (8points)
- ✧ Do you rarely eat grains such as brown rice, wild rice, buckwheat, quinoa, amaranth or millet? (10 points)

- ✧ Does your diet consist mainly of carbohydrates, especially simple ones (potatoes, bread, pasta, etc...)? (10 points)
- ✧ Do you consume alcoholic beverages regularly? (10 points)
- ✧ Are you addicted to coffee? (10 points)
- ✧ Are you overweight? (10 points)
- ✧ Do you have a lot of food allergies? (10 points)
- ✧ Do you eat pork regularly? (10 points)
- ✧ Do you eat beef regularly? (5 points)
- ✧ Do you drink diet soft drinks regularly? (15 points)
- ✧ Do you have binges of particular foods? (15 points)
- ✧ Do you have an increased intake of raw food (salad bars)? (12 points)

d. Exterior factors

Have you ever been subjected to:

- ✧ Operations (5 points)
- ✧ Intake of cytostatica (anti-cancer medication), radiation (5 points)

Have you ever taken:

- ✧ Antibiotics, especially broad-spectrum (Keflex, Bactrim, Ampicillin) (10 points)
- ✧ Tetracycline for treatment of acne (15 points)
- ✧ Birth control pills (8 points)
- ✧ Cortisone, orally or in the form of injection (15 points)

✧ Have you used or are using marijuna, cocaine or heroin? (15 points)

✧ Do you smoke? (10 points)

✧ Have you had recurrent viral or bacterial infection - more than 6 in a year? (10 points)

Are your symptoms worse:

✧ When you are exposed to ragweed / pollen? (5 points)

✧ When you rake dry leaves? (5 points)

✧ When you are in a damp basement? (5 points)

✧ Do you increasingly feel more uncomfortable with your environment (reacting to smoke, fumes, perfumes, pesticides, inability to visit public places)? (10 points)

Are you subjected to any of the following chemical stressors in your home? (5 points each)

✧ Aluminum pots and pans

✧ Amonia

✧ Fluoridated water

✧ Dyes

✧ Gas stoves

✧ Hair sprays

✧ Kerosene

✧ Lacquer

✧ Teflon pots and pans

- Turpentine
- Paint fumes
- Newspaper print
- Nail polish
- Pesticides
- Tobacco smoke
- Formaldehyde
- Are you living or have you ever lived in a damp climate for at least one year (foggy beach, damp states such as New York, Florida, Oregon or Washington D.C.)? (10 points)
- Have you ever experienced adverse reactions to any medications or drugs? (5 points)

Do the following items make you feel in any way emotionally or physically ill? (5 points each)

- Mold, mildew
- Dust
- Cats, dogs
- Gas
- Cigarettes
- Bleaches
- Paint
- Dyes
- Gasoline

- Insecticides

Do you work in a building with (5 points each):

- Inadequate lighting
- Inadequate windows present in your working area
- Recycled air
- Parking underneath the building
- Ceilings containing asbestos
- Regular lighting (absence of full spectrum lights)
- Smoking permitted
- Many copying machines, X-ray equipment or computers present?

B. SYMPTOMS

Grade the symptoms according to severity:

Occasional	: 2 points
Moderate	: 4 points
Severe	: 6 points

a. Brain symptoms

- Difficulty in concentration
- Decreased memory
- Drowsiness
- Headaches

- ✧ Severe mood swings
- ✧ Depression
- ✧ Suicidal thoughts
- ✧ Anger and irritability
- ✧ Frustration
- ✧ Defensivness, even when it is not warranted

b. Hormonal symptoms

- ✧ PMS
- ✧ Flare up of yeast infections the week before the menstrual cycle or immediatly after intercourse
- ✧ Loss of sexual desire
- ✧ Impotence
- ✧ Endometriosis
- ✧ Menstrual irregularities
- ✧ Early menopause

c. Digestive symptoms

- ✧ Gas
- ✧ Abdominal distention
- ✧ Diarrhea
- ✧ Constipation
- ✧ Hemorrhoids

- ✧ Abdominal pain
- ✧ Mucus in the stool
- ✧ Greenish stools
- ✧ Anal itching
- ✧ Heartburn
- ✧ Bad breath
- ✧ Constant hungry feeling
- ✧ Weight loss or gain without a change of diet
- ✧ Presence of a thick, yellow fur in the middle of the tongue, especially in the morning
- ✧ Food allergies

d. Other symptoms

- ✧ Recurrent colds
- ✧ Recurrent sore throats and swollen glands
- ✧ Fatigue
- ✧ Sneezing spells
- ✧ Hay fever
- ✧ Postnasal drip
- ✧ Cold limbs
- ✧ Joint and muscle pain
- ✧ Itching

- Hives
- Runny nose
- Earaches
- Hoarsness
- Intermittent fever
- Dizziness
- Watery eyes
- Blurred vision
- Mucus in bronchial tubes
- Chronic "sinusitis"
- Wheezing
- Nocturnal sweats
- Bizarre dreams
- Early morning fatigue
- Attacks of faintness

2

CEBV
OR CHRONIC EPSTEIN-BARR VIRUS

"The Yuppie Flu Strikes Again," "EB or Not EB -- That is The Question," "Journey into Fear -- The Growing Nightmare of EBV," "Stealthy Epidemic of Exhaustion," "A Disease of the Up-and-coming," "Malaise of the '80s," "Raggedy Ann Town..." Are you inundated by all these titles in various magazines and newspapers? Are all these articles overly pessimistic, and lacking in hope? Since EBV is a virus, non-holistic doctors will tell you that there is no cure. In fact, what most of those articles do, in spite of their best intentions, is to kill any hope in those suffering from this condition. In this chapter, I will explain the causes, symptoms, diagnosis and various therapeutic modalities available. I will also cite original research and personal accounts of successful treatment proving that the battle against this virus is not a hopeless one. To lose hope, is to play into the hands of this stubborn enemy, to surrender before you even start to fight.

The prevalence of "incurable" viral conditions -- EBV, CMV or Cytomegalo Virus, HTLV or HIV or the AIDS virus -- has spurred a new interest in these very ancient enemies. A better understanding of these tiny invaders will help explain difficulties we encounter in diagnosis as well as therapy.

1. VIRUSES: WHAT ARE THEY?

The word "virus" is of Latin origin and was used in ancient times to denote a noxious agent or poison. Before the discovery of filterable viruses, the word "virus" was frequently used to designate any infectious microbe irrespective of its nature. It was evident to pioneer investigators such as Edward Jenner and Louis Pasteur that disease could be caused by several classes of harmful agents. However, it soon became obvious that there were many infectious diseases which were not caused by bacteria, toxins or poisons. Eventually agents of this type were given the name of filterable viruses and later, simply, viruses.

Today, these tiny invaders are responsible for a large share of human suffering. Scientists now know that viruses cause AIDS, common colds, flu, chicken pox, measles, warts, shingles, gastroenteritis and -- EBV. Viruses are known to cause at least one form of human cancer (Burkitt's Lymphoma) and are prime suspects in several other kinds of malignancies. Yet nobody had ever seen one of those viruses even as late as 1920. That had to wait until 1931, when, with the invention of the elecronic microscope by Physicist Ernst Ruska, we at last had a clear view of the bizarre world of viruses. Multiple forms appeared before our eyes: football shapes, soccer balls, spherical, lunar shapes... but all magnificent little structures. Nothing is wasted: each one is simply a core of genetic material -- either a DNA or RNA molecule -- surrounded by a protective protein shell. Unlike other creatures, the virus cannot metabolize nutrients, in other words, cannot feed itself. It depends entirely on the help of the host, which makes it the ultimate parasite. What it does is insert its genes into the DNA of the host cell. Once activated, the viral genes order the cell to begin producing more viruses, carbon copies of the original invader. Without the help of the host, it cannot multiply itself.

Although acute viral infections like influenza kill thousands of people each year -- especially the elderly and children -- most people are able to defeat these tiny invaders. Fever, chills, swollen lymph nodes, and itchy rashes are due to the vigorous activity of the immune system, in a merciless battle with these viruses. Other viruses have a different approach. Between attacks, they will lie dormant in the body, waiting like vultures to reactivate in moments of when the host's immune system is suppressed. Herpes Simplex Viruses are a good example of this tactic. The hiding places are different: the Herpes Zoster, which causes chicken pox, sometimes hides in nerve cells and causes -

- years after the pox attack -- the excruciating attack of shingles. The Epstein-Barr virus, or Herpes Simplex III, hides in the B-cells, the very cells that make antibodies to viruses. It is the Trojan horse in the body!

Medical researchers are currently trying to make vaccinations from restructered viruses, thereby creating remedies, so desperately needed in the battle against viral diseases. But viruses have the ability to change in structure constantly creating mutations that can escape the killing effect of the vaccines.

2. "EB OR NOT EB," THAT'S THE QUESTION!

Medical experts are struggling, often with limited success, to understand a "mysterious" illness that leaves its victims exhausted months or years at a time. The ailment, known as Chronic Epstein-Barr Virus Infection, has stirred rising concern in public and medical circles for years. What is this EBV, and is it a new virus?

Not at all. The EB virus has been known for quite a while, since its discovery by Epstein and Barr, two medical researchers. It is known that the same virus causes Mononucleosis Infectiosa, more commonly known as the "Mono" or "Kissing Disease." Mono hits the young population, especially in overcrowded places such as schools and army barracks and gets its name -- "Kissing Disease" -- from the way the virus is transmitted: through droplet infection. Therefore, about 80% of the population has antibodies against the EB virus. Young people affected by mono usually suffer from extreme fatigue, sore throats and swollen, painful neck lymph nodes, pretty much part of the picture we see in the present epidemic of CEBV (Chronic Epstein-Barr Virus). It lasts about 4 to 6 weeks, before the immune system takes over and suppresses the virus.

Less known among the general population is the fact that this same virus causes two more dangerous conditions: nasopharyngeal cancer (affecting the nose and throat), especially in the Far East, and Burkitt's Lymphoma, a form of leukemia, occurring in Central Africa. Very little is known about the mechanism of EB in these two cancer forms, but attention was drawn to the Burkitt's Lymphoma connection by a frightening story here in the United States.

It started in March, 1983. Within a period of three months, four family members, living in different areas of the United States contracted non-Hodgkin's Lymphoma, a cancer of the immune system. What at first seemed unbelievable had to be accepted later: they "caught" cancer from a 63-year-old aunt visiting them from South Africa in 1982. The aunt had suffered from a severe sore throat during her tour, and the family wondered if she had somehow passed along an infection that caused cancer. While medical investigators could not find any link to a viral cause of non-Hodgkin's Lymphoma, they found that Burkitt's Lymphoma, which especially affects black African children, is strongly associated with the Epstein-Barr virus.

Four of the twelve relatives the aunt visited showed signs of recent EB infection, while one of the cancer victims also showed signs of EB. The two other victims tested negative, while the fourth victim died before testing was done. The aunt had become ill just before she left Africa, which might suggest the possibility that some variation of EB virus, or maybe a totally different virus, was responsible for this cancer cluster. In the meantime a second victim has died, while the other two are in remission.

My opinion is that only four out of the twelve relatives got non-Hodgkin's Lymphoma because the disease (virus or bacteria) was only able to penetrate the immune systems of four. It would be very interesting to find out whether these four victims had recently gone through emotional and/or physical hardships, severe enough to suppress their immune systems allowing a cancer form to develop down the road. They also might have had other viral infections roaming through their bodies at the same time, such as Herpes Simplex I or II (the sexual form); or Candida might have weakened their immune system enough, allowing this perverse unknown invader to do its damage.

The suggestion of a new agent working in tandem with the EB virus was proposed. One of the suspects is HBLV, a newly discovered herpes virus. Could HBLV be the unidentified transmissible agent in both cases? Like the EB virus, it infects B-cells, is associated with cancer, and is prevalent in certain regions of Africa. Robert Gallo, whose National Cancer Institute lab discovered HBLV, confirms that blood samples from some of the South African's relatives have tested positive for HBLV. The key to the solution is the analysis of the aunt herself. Naturally, all this negative publicity has made a lonely soul of this victim, since friends have been avoiding her. Small wonder that the woman refuses to cooperate with further investigations.

In view of these three possible different pictures, Mononucleosis, nasopharyngeal cancer and Burkitt's Lymphoma, all caused by the infamous EB virus, why would it be impossible to have our fourth actual clinical syndrome present -- Chronic Epstein-Barr Virus? Doctors react very differently towards this EB diagnosis. Some call it the latest health hysteria or the fad of the decade; others, such as Dr. Anthony Komaroff, Director of the Department of General Medicine at Brigham and Women's hospital, in Boston, whose group has studied more than 500 patients suffering from the syndrome, realize that it can be unquestionably devastating to those affected. Others call it "an epidemic of diagnosis," meaning that doctors are overdiagnosing the disease, making it a catch-all explanation for symptoms that otherwise cannot be explained.

Still others think that "a lot of illness associated with CEBV is probably ordinary neuroses which are manifested as tiredness. It's a disease mostly of younger adults who are having problems in what are ordinarily difficult phases of life. These people are very unhappy, and it's often hard to sort out how many of their psychological problems come from their illness and how many cause their illness." Some doctors contend that these patients only "look for a relationship with their physician and want to find, at any cost, a physical cause of their illness." A few physicians believe that this EBV picture is not new at all, that what these patients complain of has been recognized for over a century. These doctors are also convinced that this syndrome is not expanding.

Perhaps what we medical professionals should do before passing judgment on a whole group of patients is to sit back and listen to what they have to say.

The "malaise" may be said to have begun in Incline Village, Nevada, on the north shore of Lake Tahoe, in 1985. Of course, it was not the start of the EBV epidemic; it was rather the first time attention was drawn towards a mysterious illness, striking a small town in epidemic proportions with symptoms of Mononucleosis--swollen glands, sore throats, aching muscles. But there was a difference: unlike mononucleosis, the symptoms would not go away. One woman described herself as feeling like a Raggedy Ann doll, without the stuffing; other individuals who were able to run marathons one day were not able to walk two miles without being exhausted the next. Some became total recluses, isolated from family and friends, who were afraid of catching this "bug." They, themselves, were too tired to go to social gatherings, theaters or simply their jobs. Sufferers described it as living in a nightmare that never ends. A few compared it to AIDS. This is almost inevitable when one mentions the malaise of the '80s. But the differences are more pronounced. For one thing, AIDS kills; chronic Mono, as one patient puts it, "just makes you wish you were dead."

Many EBV patients are devastated by the skepticism of their doctors and friends. "After a while you feel better and you start questioning yourself. You try to do some work, two hours here, one hour there -- and pay the penalty for the entire next week! It's like riding a roller coaster." Most victims' lives revolve around two things: work (because they have to for economic reasons) and rest. They spell it out: "There is no F-U-N."

The symptoms that drives EBV sufferers really crazy is "brain fog" which leads to difficulty in concentrating, or remembering the simplest things. It has been compared to "having endless mononucleosis with a touch of Alzheimer." Others feel relieved when a diagnosis is made, even one as bad as cancer: at least their suffering is "validated" in people's eyes, and CEBV was killing their spirit more than their body.

Is it conceivable that all these people, at one point enjoying healthy and active lives, change overnight, because they are "neurotic," "unhappy," "bored," "crave attention" or "lazy?" Hardly. This idea is simply an insult to the millions of those who suffer! I feel extra compassion for these victims who draw little sympathy from friends and doctors. We do have here a new epidemic caused by a debilitating disease.

Much of the problem is probably the result of the name. The medical community relies too much on names to describe conditions and, therefore, gets tangled up in attempts to diagnose new variations. After calling the disorder CEBV, the doctor turns to his textbook of twenty years ago, and he finds Mono, nasopharyngeal cancer and Burkitt's Lymphoma, as the diseases caused by this virus. The medical community is slow to recognize that the EB virus can cause yet another syndrome. Therefore, it fails to take into consideration the enormous changes that have take place in our general environment, food intake, and normal emotional stress, as outlined in the first chapter.

It is quite possible that an EB-related virus will be found to have caused the "malaise of the '80s." Once the real agent is found, (and in my opinion it will be a mixture of viruses and yeast cells), the disease will certainly be renamed. Australia and New Zealand did not wait to do just that. They found names such as CEBV or Post-Viral Fatigue unsuitable and called the condition "Myalgic-Encephalitic Syndrome" or "M.E.S.," describing the muscle-and-brain symptoms. But whatever the eventual name, these sufferers need immediate attention -- a name alone has never been a guarantee of a cure. Our Western medical lexicon is full of the most exotic names, and yet mostly they describe incurable conditions with unknown etiologies. Do we desert those people, too?

3. CEBV, A DISEASE OF THE YUPPIES?

"A disease of the up-and-coming" and "Yuppie Flu" are terms consistently used and heard when CEBV is mentioned. This has some pejorative connotations in most people's minds, as if the condition were one of the fad attributes of ambitious young persons. What's the reason? Do actively striving people deserve to be looked upon as neurotic overachievers, falling back on a fashionable disease to explain their frustrations and daily tensions?

There is no doubt that CEBV is found mainly among people in their early 30s and 40s, predominantly females. The victims are typically extra vigorous. They do more exercise, have more social life and are more successful in their careers than the average person. This hardly sounds like a class of hypochondriacs!

There is an explanation for this "yuppie" syndrome. First of all, the fact that it hits more women than men is a myth. The reason is that men are diagnosed less often is because they visit their doctors less often. This holds true also for any other ailment (migraine, arthritis, depression, etc.) Men simply deal differently with common symptoms such as fatigue, headaches, mood swings, muscle pains. They tend not to take time off when these generalized symptoms appear, but rather blame tensions at work, too much beer intake, too much food, a fight with their spouses, anything but the possibility of some bug penetrating their defense system. It is the usual "macho" picture.

Secondly, it is called the yuppie disease because a disproportionate number of its victims have been young, white professionals. Hollywood is alleged to be plagued by the disease. But on the other hand, people between 30 and 40 have been exposed the longest to all recently emerging factors that suppress our immune system. As discussed in Chapter One, our problem started in 1940 with the introduction of antibiotics, later aggravated by changes in our food, cortisone, the pill, and, finally by the tremendous pressure we put on ourselves emotionally to be successful.

One is classified as a failure if one does not own a vacation house, a luxury car which is the status symbol and a professional job with a good pension plan. I am not shooting such achievements down as worthless, but it is disenchanting to see this become the exclusive goal for many young people. Closeness to nature, to family and friends is often forgotten, people are simply too busy making a living. The young people in schools already feel the pressure: the accent is on career, the stock market and how to be young, successful entrepreneurs. I am convinced that many among them are hit by the onset of CEBV, because exposure for 15-20 years to all the known triggering factors is enough to suppress the immune system, allowing a reactivation of EB already present in the body or the invasion of new enemies.

That CEBV hits the high achievers harder than anybody else is normal, because the stress factor is probably the biggest insult to our immune system. The mind-body connection (see page # 61) deserves a lot more attention in the pathogenesis of disease than it has received until now. I have seen that in most of the immune-suppressed diseases (Candida, CEBV, Herpes Simplex I & II), an emotional upset is the major triggering factor for relapse and reactivation of viruses.

As doctor and confidant to our patients, it is our duty to be part of their support group. Just knowing that they have a diagnosable disorder helps them to ease the depression. We should not prolong and stimulate more despair in these patients by giving them the merry-go-round treatment of the medical field. We must avoid the endless hospitalizations and tests, that take place while doctors try vainly to find out what is wrong with them. We also have to think of the humiliation patients experience when they return to work after bouts of CEBV because they are not able to tell co-workers what has been wrong with them. We doctors have to take their plight seriously. As one of my patients expressed it: "There is a whole segment of the medical profession that says it doesn't exist; I wish they had it."

4. EPIDEMIOLOGY AND MECHANISM OF SPREADING

Epstein-Barr virus is a member of the herpes family viruses, which causes chicken pox, cold sores, genital lesions, shingles, and other ailments. All these viruses are tricky. As already mentioned, they have the habit of hiding out in the body in a latent state; then they get reactivated and attack. But even in this elusive company, the Epstein-Barr virus stands out as the most eccentric and fascinating herpes of them all. Perhaps more is known about EBV infection in man than any other herpes virus-host interaction.

Investigations have shown that EBV is widely disseminated throughout the world. The key epidemiological fact about the virus is that it shows up everywhere. Blood samples collected from isolated tribes in the Amazon rain forests have proved free of measles antibodies but positive for Epstein-Barr. The virus is easily passed along in the saliva, which explains its ubiquity.

Oddly enough, the consequences of contracting the virus vary dramatically from place to place and culture to culture. In the United States and Europe, it causes the "kissing disease" or Mono; in Africa, it is involved with Burkitt's Lymphoma, a fast-growing tumor of the jaw, promptly leading to death. EBV seems to be also closely implicated with Kaposi's Sarcoma and multiple sclerosis. In Asia, the same virus has been linked to nasopharyngeal cancer.

Why would this same virus lead to all these different clinical results? Part of the answer lies in the company of what we can call "co-factors." Burkitt's Lymphoma, for example, appears in a belt across central Africa marked by high rainfall and warm temperatures -- the precise features of mosquito country. The co-factor allowing the virus to trigger Burkitt's Lymphoma seems to be a weakening of the immune system brought on by constant exposure to malaria and yellow fever, and as we mentioned in Chapter one, **humidity** is **the** climatic factor that weakens the immune system.

In the case of Mono, the key co-factor is age. In general, a toddler exposed to the Epstein-Barr virus will develop antibodies and never exhibit so much as a sniffle. An older child may have a mild sore throat for a day or two. But a young adult encountering the virus for the first time stands a better than even chance of spending a truly miserable month in bed with Mono. Obviously if early exposure to the virus confers a kind of immunity, conventional ideas about hygiene don't hold up. In Indonesia and Mexico, where nearly all children have the EB virus in their bloodstream by age six, infectious mononucleosis is unheard of. But in Sweden or England, where parents are fastidious about kissing, many infants and young children don't get exposed; as a result they develop Mono as teenagers.

This viral omnipresence helps explain why the Center for Disease Control (CDC) and doctors are so leery of reports of widespread new epidemics of EBV. After all, you can hardly have an epidemic of a disease when everybody already has antibodies in his or her bloodstream. Or can you? I think we fail to understand the co-factors involved in this CEBV epidemic. For one, the common root is the suppressed immune system, the triggering factors of which I have extensively discussed in the first chapter. Another co-factor is the concomitant presence of the other Herpes Simplex viruses in patients, H. Simplex I (cold sores), H. Simplex II (genital herpes) and H. Simplex IV or CMV (Cytomegalovirus).

Latent presence with occasional flare-ups of these viruses are continous onslaughts against the strength of the immune system, exhausting it to a level where the EB virus can creep upon you without warning. Perhaps the least understood and accepted cofactor, but in my opinion one of the most important, is the presence of Candida Albicans, a common yeast cell.This microorganism is extensively discussed in the next chapter. In common practice I have seen that even for patients with confirmed EBV, Candida was present well before the EBV could attack. Knowing the insidious character of Candida cells, which sense a small drop in the strength of your immune system long before any laboratory test can detect it, we can conclude that Candida should always be suspected when we have an EB patient in our office.

How does the EB virus pull all those tricks on us? This is best explained at the cellular level. It is known that the virus infects the B lymphocytes of the immune system, our white blood cells formed in the bone marrow that normally manufacture antibodies against disease. Once infected by the virus, the B-cells proliferate lustily and become immortalized. As mentioned in Chapter One, the response of our immune system is the production of a legion of activated Killer T cells. During the course of the infection, the patient feels horribly sick, since the immune system is literally at war with itself. It is this "Herxheimer reaction," the formation of toxins, that puzzles the patient at first. Are we not used to getting **immediate** positive results from our "magic bullets?" We take a sleeping pill and we eventually fall asleep. It is extremely important that the patient understands that the process of getting well at the microbial level temporarily makes him feel sicker than ever. This is the case for every immune-suppressed disease.

The threat of EBV is never wholly eliminated, however. A few transformed B-cells harboring the virus -- about one in a million -- remain present in otherwise healthy individuals. It is like a slow, incessant battle between T-cells and a few virus-infected B-cells, neither party claiming victory. The primary infection occurs by the oral route. There is, however, growing evidence that the primary site of viral replication is not in the B lymphocytes but in the pharynx. Infectious virus particles can be regularly found in the throat washings of Mono patients. Moreover, small amounts of virus have been regularly detected in the saliva of approximately 20% of healthy blood positive patients. Random surveys of previously infected individuals have suggested that at any given time a significant portion (25%) are shedding infectious virus into the throat. You can see the enormous importance of how this virus gets transmitted via saliva or kisses to immune-suppressed patients. And with virtually all previously infected healthy individuals thus far analysed, a surprisingly high frequency of specific memory cells can be found in their blood. This really means that there is a continuous war-truce going on, a state of high alert, easily erupting into a full-fledged battle when the co-factors discussed above intervene.

5. SYMPTOMS

One of the problems for doctors in confirming a diagnosis of EBV is the variety and non-specificness of the symptoms. Who has never suffered from fatigue, some depression, muscle pain? To make matters worse, another epidemic, Candida, has many of the same symptoms. But to really confound the doctor, both conditions exist simultaneously in 75% of the cases. Of course, we always have our laboratory tests to help distinguish between the two conditions. Notice that I said, "help;" in no way are lab tests the deciding factor. Clinically, however, we can distinguish between Candida and EBV, if both don't exist together. This will be shown in Chapter Three, on Candida.

What symptoms are we looking for in the case of EBV? There is a group of **Key Symptoms**, which should be present at some time during the course of the illness:

Relapsing, intermittent character of the symptoms.

Exhaustion.

Muscle pain or weakness upon exercising.

Unusual muscle fatigue.

A history of illness lasting more than three months.

Besides these key symptoms, there is a group of common symptoms, which can, but don't have to, exist at some time during the course of the disease. Often patients and doctors mistakenly conclude that if the patients have not had sore throats, they can't possibly have EBV.

COMMON SYMPTOMS

"Brain fog": inability to concentrate and remember simple things. Some individuals have to read a passage three times before it makes sense to them. Patients forget the name of their friends, they go to another room to pick something up and forget what it is by the time they get there. What is also distressing is that this brain fog fluctuates in character. Victims never know when it is going to hit them, which creates much anxiety, especially when it occurs in professional people with a high degree of responsibility. This brain "damage" will express itself, too, in a lack of coordination, excessive drowsiness and balance disturbance. If we did not know better, we would diagnose them as "Alzheimer" victims.

How to explain these symptoms? There are two observations that give us the answer, one found in Traditional Chinese Medicine, the other in our latest modern technology. Chinese medicine considers the spleen-pancreas organ also as "the sea of marrow" or seat of memory. Those doctors look at this entity (they called it the "I") as a filing cabinet full of little drawers where data is stored, ready to be checked out the moment we need it. We have fully explained in Chapter One that the spleen-pancreas is the immune system. A decrease in the strength of this organ will affect every functional aspect of it -- hence the memory is decreased.

Closer observations in our time have also disclosed some disturbing events. After the first documented outbreak of CEBV in Lake Tahoe, repeated CAT scans of the victims brains showed bright white spots, somewhat like the spots found in multiple sclerosis, but smaller. It is a fact that many neurologists now observe bright white spots on CAT scans, which they appropriately named "UBO's" or "Unidentified Bright Objects." It is my conviction that many of those patients, if not all, suffer from EBV. It is just a matter of time before a neurologist will look into this matter.

It is interesting that the location of the spots on the brain correspond closely to the patient's neurological symptoms, identically as they would in Multiple Sclerosis. For instance, a bright spot in the Capsula Interna of the brain would yield parestesia, numbness and decreased strength in the upper/lower extremity. There is a danger in this picture: it is a distinct possibility that patients diagnosed as having MS are actually suffering from EBV, the latter a condition we can cure. Imagine the despair of victims when they hear a diagnosis as dreadful as MS, when in fact a more treatable condition is the cause. We must not forget that there is no test available to prove with 100% accuracy that somebody suffers from MS!

In other words, every respectable neurologist should eliminate in his first differential diagnosis of MS, CEBV -- particularly as it now exists in epidemic proportions. Ruling out CEBV before throwing a patient into depression with a diagnosis of MS is an act of compassion, responsibility and professionalism. And to all the potential victims of MS: it would be wise to first rule out CEBV before you accept the final diagnosis of MS, especially when only one attack has occurred.

Muscle symptom: muscle twitching and delayed muscle recovery. Muscle tenderness.

Infectious symptoms: recurrent sore throats, recurrent colds and painful lymph nodes in the neck.

Psychological symptoms: depression and severe mood swings -- one can feel fine at 10 a.m., yet be totally depressed at 2 p.m. This does not create a lot of sympathy on the part of family and friends, who do not understand what is going on. In fact, most relatives and associates become upset with this behavior, which can lead to disrupted marriages, other relationships and friendships. Exactly **not** what a CEBV patient needs. Anger and irritability are other common symptoms. Of course, the lack of support from family and doctors only adds fuel to the fire, completing the vicious circle: the patient is now in an even more dangerous state of all-consuming anger and despair.

Gastrointestinal symptoms: I believe that these symptoms are minimal in the CEBV patient; if present, a diagnosis of CANDIDA should be ruled out first. Symptoms such as irritable bowel syndrome, gas, distension and constipation are more likely linked to a generalized yeast infection.

6. DIAGNOSIS

The cornerstone of diagnosis has to be the clinical picture. As discussed above, the diagnosis can become complicated clinically because of symptoms in common with other immune-suppressed diseases (Candida, Parasites, CMV, AIDS). This is not unusual. We have to remember that all these diseases have a common root: the suppressed immune system. It is like riding on a freeway: at the entrance, for Candida, CEBV, CMV -- at the exit, for cancer, leukemia and AIDS. The symptoms have to be similar, since all these conditions are derived from the same starting point. Only the intensity differs. This being the case, it is somewhat helpful to be able to fall back on laboratory tests that are available. I have learned in my practice that many doctors, when they ask for the EBV test, are still unable to give a correct interpretation of the results. What I want to do here therefore is explain the interpretation of the different antibody formations in the case of EBV infections.

EBV antibody titers (levels) are tests indicating the body's response to EBV antigens, which are complex substances produced by the virus during different stages of replication. The immune system recognizes antigens as being foreign. Once EBV enters the body, its antigens stimulate the production of antibodies -- proteins carried in the blood to respond to infection.

Although laboratories performing these tests present the results in slightly different ways, the titers are recorded in four parts:

VCA-IgG or Viral Capsid Antigen

EAD or Early Antigen Diffuse Component

EAR or Early Antigen Restricted Component

EBNA or Epstein-Barr Nuclear Antigen

The titer value of EBV antibody may be written as a ratio, such as 1:320. The interpretation of EBV antibody titers is based on the following premises:

1. Once a person becomes infected with EBV, the anti-VCA antibodies appear first.

2. Anti-EA antibodies appear next, or are present with anti-VCA antibodies early in the course of illness. Titers higher than those seen in people who have recovered from infection and have no symptoms indicate active disease. An anti-EA antibody titer >80 (>=greater than) in someone 2 years after primary infection is the current working level of diagnosis.

3. As the patient recovers, anti-VCA and anti-EA antibodies decrease, and anti-EBNA antibodies appear. Anti-EBNA reflects a past infection.

4. After the patient is well, anti-VCA and anti-EBNA are always present. These titers persist for life, but usually in lower ranges than those appearing in acute illness.

The above findings are reflected in Table # 5

What do we see in CEBV?

EBV-VCA-IgG antibody 1:640 or higher

Low or absent anti-VCA IgM

EAD detectable, for instance 1:80

EAR detectable, for instance <10

EBNA relatively low compared with the IgG, for instance 40

Most likely because of the complexity of the test, another variation was introduced: A IgG titer of >1.10 means positive for EBV; a value higher than 3.40 is "high positive."

Other worthwile tests to be done are antibody titers against Coxsackie B viruses, since they seem to play a role in the pathogenesis of CEBV. Very frequently high antibody titers (>512) are found in CEBV patients.

Another test is the determination of the T4/T8 Ratio, part of our "Immune Panel." Often we see a reduction in the ratio and a

Table # 5

ANTIBODY RESPONSES TO EBV-INDUCED INFECTIOUS MONONUCLEOSIS

	IgG (VCA) (Chronic)	IgM (VCA) (Acute)	EA (Acute)	EBNA
Detectable in acute phase	yes	yes	yes	
Appears at 1-6 months				yes
Persists for life	yes			yes

significant reduction in the numbers of suppressor cells in an acutely ill group.

7. THERAPY

One of the things that doctors hate about EBV is the fact that they feel hopeless in bringing any relief to patients. I think this was one of the reasons that it took doctors so long to acknowledge the syndrome. I still often hear from my patients: "My doctor thought maybe EBV might play a role, but even if it did, we could not really do anything about it." "Go home, rest and hope that it will pass soon," is another frequently heard statement. Not very encouraging to people who live in a daze, shell-shocked from a condition that seems to come out of a clear blue sky. One day they were healthy, the next they were only a fraction of their usual selves. What I will discuss in this section are the different current treatments with their pros and cons.

a. REST

Never has this advice been given so frequently to a specific class of patients. Do these victims feel too tired to put one foot in front of the other? It seems a logical step that rest is the best advice we can give them. I think this is completely wrong. Don't misunderstand me. I know these people are tired; but think for a moment. Have you ever sat on your sofa all day watching TV or stayed in bed, doing nothing? How will you feel at the end of such a day? Even if you are completely healthy, you will feel very tired! It is simple: non-movement means stagnation, including stagnation of your energy. Nothing will work properly anymore and all the organs will start functioning at 50% of their strength, creating a real "back-up," closing a vicious circle of lassitude and causing a feeling of heaviness. I am not saying EBV patients should prepare for the next Olympic Games; rather they should take at least a half hour's light exercise daily, consisting of swimming, walking or biking. It is interesting to see that even when patients feel they cannot move their limbs, they feel better after the exercise. Patients should avoid weight lifting: this simply will be too strenuous.

The best time to do this exercise is right at the beginning of the day, even before breakfast. By getting rid of toxins accumulated during the night, you will benefit from early perspiration the whole day!

b. SINEQUAN

Sinequan is a tricyclic antidepressant with potent antihistaminic and anti-inflammatory effects. Usually the dosage is at least 40 mg. The dosage used for these patients is usually 10 mg taken at night. A few patients find relief with this method. I wonder how many symptoms it really masks and whether or not the patients simply feel better because it makes them feel less depressed. Personally, I have discovered that it only seems to help in about 10% of the cases and only for a short time.

c. TAGAMET (CIMETIDINE)

The topselling medication in many countries, but not for EBV reasons. It is a potent medication for any stomach disorder, especially ulcers. How was this introduced in EBV treatment? Researchers observed that very young children, who have no Suppressor T-cells, often have no symptoms when they have an EBV infection. Suppressor T-cells have receptors for Cimetidine, which would decrease their function. By taking this drug, some patients showed some improvement. However, the symptoms seemed to come back after the therapy was stopped. A similar pattern was found with Zantac, which also had to be taken indefinitely.

d. ACYCLOVIR (ZOVIRAX)

It was the first available approved antiviral drug in 1985. The main indication was the battle against Herpes Simplex II or Genital Herpes. Since EBV belongs to the family of Herpes Simplex viruses, some researchers tried to use it for CEBV. However, the drug seems to have very little effect on the EB virus. It is an expensive drug, and in my opinion, it is a waste of time and money to use it for CEBV.

e. INJECTIONS

Holistic and nutritionally oriented doctors have found the benefit of vitamin therapy. The first indicated is Vitamin C, and there is no doubt that Vitamin C, given in an intravenous push or drip, will benefit the patient. Linus Pauling, the father of Vitamin C therapy, advises doses orally up to 30,000 mgs if tolerated (loose stools indicates the patient should cut back). Another proven energy stimulus with these patients is injections with Disiccated Liver, Folic Acid, AMP and Panthothenic Acid (B12). Two injections a week for several weeks will help EBV sufferers.

Although some provide modest improvement, the above therapies do not look too promising. There is good news on the horizon however: 1) a specific diet (discussed in Chapter six) and 2) a newly discovered therapy with herbal products, discussed in Chapter eight.

8. FREQUENTLY HEARD QUESTIONS

1. Is CEBV contagious?

Most likely one has already been exposed to the EB virus. Whether one develops CEBV, a chronic condition, depends on how one's body deals with the virus. Those in close contact with CEBV patients do not seem to develop CEBV any more frequently than anyone else. Patients suffering from CEBV should not bear sole responsibility for spreading the disease. Every individual is responsible for maintaining his own strong immune system, avoiding any penetration by a virus. It is a good idea for CEBV patients tients not to come in close contact with severely immune-suppressed patients (cancer, Candida, etc.). However, many do not develop the illness at all even after exposure. The ability to resist is directly related to the presence of a strong immune system. In general CEBV is harder to catch than the flu, chicken pox or Herpes Simplex. It takes intimate contact -- kissing, or sharing of eating utensils, for example.

2. What causes the infection to flare up repeatedly?

Any of the triggering factors reducing or decreasing the strength of the immune system can cause a flare-up. The intermittent course of the disease is a perfect reflection of the battle between the virus and the immune system defenders. Low-grade fevers are commonly present and are also signs of this battle.

3. Are there any support groups?

There is a support group for EBV patients, located in Portland, Oregon, at the following address:

National CEBV Syndrome Association, Inc.
P.O. Box 230108
Portland, OR 97223
(503) 684-5261

9. CMV (CYTOMEGALOVIRUS)

Cytomegalovirus is a major human pathogen. It also belongs to the Herpes Simplex family and is called Herpes Simplex 4. It is clear that CMV is responsible for significant medical problems. It is especially feared during pregnancy, where it is a major factor in congenital retardation. However, it is frequently found in people with a positive CEBV titer and can be presumed to be a cofactor in the symptomatology of the CEBV syndrome. There is a constant potential for flare-ups. Once infected with CMV we harbor the virus within our cells for life and are always at some risk of recurrence of CMV infection. That is exactly what happens with victims of a suppressed immune system. Often when blood tests are done -- antibody tests such as in EBV -- high titers are found in conjunction with high titers of EBV, Herpes Simplex I and II. In the Western medical world, prospects for treatment are not as bright as methods for prevention of CMV disease at the present time. The only drug now available that has any chance of being effective is Acyclovir. But even in the most optimistic opinion, it is only marginally active against CMV.

The more promising therapy, again, is the therapy with herbal products combined with the diet as outlined for EBV. Titers can be brought back to normal with the disappearance of most of the symptoms.

10. SOCIO-ECONOMIC CONSEQUENCES OF EBV/CMV

Looking at the living hell patients have to go through, it is not unusual that they cannot keep on working. No matter what the job is, brainfog, fatigue and muscle pain can influence any task negatively. Going on disability, frustrating for these young people, is the only solution. Only then can they pay attention to their recovery. But here is another major obstacle: with many doctors still not accepting this diagnosis, the "disability doctor" frequently will state in his raport that such a condition does not exist and that the patient is suffering from a "psycho-somatic disease with somatization," a nice phrase meaning that "it is all in the head, and the patient has some hysteric components" -- the latter explaining his physical symptoms.

In the "Annals of Internal Medicine", 1988, 108:387-389, an article appeared -- "Chronic Fatigue Syndrome: A working Case Definition", by Holmes et al., from the Division of Viral Diseases, Centers of Disease Control (CDC), Atlanta, Georgia. Their goal was to set up some major clinical criteria to define Chronic Fatigue Syndrome (CFS), since in their opinion, there is doubt as to the diagnostic value of positive EBV blood titers, associated with the proposed relationship between the Epstein-Barr virus infection and patients who have been diagnosed with this syndrome. They concluded (rightfully in my opinion, as I have said before) that it was premature to focus diagnostic efforts on Epstein-Barr virus alone.

The same criteria can be used for any immuno-suppressed condition, Candida included. What are those criteria?

Major Criteria

1. A new onset of debilitating fatigue in a previous healthy individual, severe enough to reduce the daily activity of the patient with at least 50% in comparison with his status before the disease.

2. Other clinical conditions with similar symptoms must be excluded at the same time. Of course this includes most of the

immuno-suppressed and auto-immune conditions already mentioned on page # 1.

Unfortunately, it exposes the patient to an expensive and not always harmless battery of tests, sometimes leading to a loss of precious time in the healing of the patient.

Minor Criteria

Most of these criteria are the symptoms of EBV mentioned before in this chapter. They include: sore throats, muscle weakness, painful lymph nodes, mild fevers, headaches, insomnia, brain fog and joint pains.

Some physical criteria are also denoted: mild fevers, pharyngitis and palpable cervial lymphnodes.

It is important for patients, forced to go on disability, to arm themselves with these criteria and present them to their doctor.

References:

"Medical Evaluation", 2-88, 24575.005, Evaluation of Chronic Epstein-Barr Virus Syndrome.

"Chronic Fatigue in Primary Care," from the Department of Medicine and Psychology, Fort Sam Houston, Texas.

"Chronic Fatigue Syndrome and the Diagnostic Utility of Antibody to Epstein-Barr Virus Early Antigen," from the Division of Infectious Diseases and Internal medicine and the section of Clinical Microbiology, Mayo Clinic, appeared in JAMA Aug 19, 88.

3

CANDIDA

1. INTRODUCTION

Just when you think that CEBV is one of the most dire threats of this decade, another enemy lurks around the corner: Candida Albicans. It is a yeastlike fungus whose habitat is the mucosae of warm blooded animals and humans. In individuals whose immune system is intact the organism is typically benign, but Candida is a better clinician and can discover slight changes in the immune system earlier in their development than we can with our chemical tests. In other words, yeast cells have slipped through an "open door" in your body to start their devastating work of multiplication before you even know that the door is open.

What is remarkable at this time is that Candida is considerably less accepted by the medical community than CEBV. It has not acquired the notoriety of CEBV, which is the topic of numerous articles in magazines and newspapers and the conversation on TV shows. However, let's not forget that it took the medical community, and the public in general, almost a decade to accept that CEBV exists and might cause some problems in certain individuals. The result is that CEBV is currently overdiagnosed to the neglect of Candida.

Why is this? Doctors now call it "the hypoglycemia" of the '80s, referring to the "epidemic" of diagnosed hypoglycemics in the '70s. Back then, much attention was drawn to a syndrome consisting of fainting attacks, with cold sweat, sudden fatigue, cold limbs, shakiness and trembling, reversed by eating some protein. The major therapeutic measure was an adjustment of the diet, eliminating sweets and prescribing more frequent, smaller meals -- five a day. Although these therapeutic measures were successful to a degree, they were still considered a "fad" that would pass. Now that Candida has come to the foreground, those critics seem to be right in their opinion.

One of the problems with doctors is that they rely too much on labels and laboratory tests. For instance, our medical world is full of fancy names for diseases that have no cure: they simply describe symptoms. Look at "PCE" or "Polyarthritis Chronica Evolutiva," or in the more popular term "Rheumatoid Arthritis." Neurology is full of those names (Amyotropic Lateral Sclerosis, Multiple Sclerosis, Olivo-Ponto-Cerebellar Atrophy, etc.). So when "Candida Albicans" emerges, most doctors return to their text books to find that Systemic Candidiasis is a "deadly disease, requiring hospitalization with intravenous administration of Amphotericine." That's what most patients will hear from their doctors when they suggest that they might be suffering from this condition. Again they are not taking into account the dramatic changes that have occurred in our environment, food intake and emotional lives, as discussed in Chapter One. Candida is present right now in people's systems in much higher amounts than we may anticipate. The total of Candida sufferers would make the numbers of CEBV victims seem minimal, because the Candida cell is a lot more clever and opportunistic than the EB virus.

Another factor causing doctors to discount Candida is that they are better acquainted with blood tests for CEBV: this test is readily requested, while Candida lab tests -- and there are several different ones -- seem to be unknown to the majority of doctors. Facing a complicated set of symptoms, most doctors may ask for a routine blood panel, which, with the exception of slight anemia, turns out to be normal. When a doctor does not consider the possibility of Candida it is unlikely that he will even ask for such a test. So the patient is told "on paper you look perfectly healthy," and -- it is implied -- there is no reason to feel sick. "Get on with your life; you are thirty now, time to get married and have some children." Of course, this merely adds insult to injury, plunging the patient into frustration and deep depression.

It is hard to believe that these tiny microflora or yeast cells, subsisting on the surface of all living things, can play such havoc with our body. Normally yeast cells live in harmony with other bacteria in a concentration of millions of bacteria versus one Candida cell. These bacteria form the normal flora of the gastro-intestinal tract and inhibit the overgrowth of yeast in normal circumstances. We will see in the next pages what triggering factors turn these innocent-looking creatures into vultures, how we can detect them, what symptoms they cause, and finally, what our most succesful battle plan will be.

2. HOW DO WE RECOGNIZE THAT WE SUFFER FROM THIS CONDITION?

The symptomatology of Candidiasis is a doctor's delight! Don't misunderstand me. It is not because the diagnosis is easy, but the broad pattern of symptoms gives each specialist in the medical field the opportunity to have a crack at this disease. That is exactly what happens. Patients consult their gynecologists for vaginal yeast infections and are prescribed antifungal cream or vaginal tablets to take. The vaginal discharge seems to disappear after 5-6 days but recurs with the next menstrual cycle or right after sexual intercourse. But no problem. A low dosage of antibiotics is now advised after each intercourse.

Then things get out of hand: after numerous further episodes of vaginal discharge, the patient is never free from this curse. The doctor cannot seem to find any cause for the condition. Oh, yes. The patient had some minor surgery just before the first attack. The surgery was complicated by an infection and logically, broad-spectrum antibiotics were prescribed intravenously for five days. And, of course, there was increasing stress at work and at home, as a result of the dual career expected of the modern woman. But it doesn't occur to the doctor that this has anything to do with those yeast infections. Finally the patient gets tired of all those vaginal creams. And frankly, it is an embarrassment for the gynecologist too. The solution is to send the patient to another specialist.

With the multiple food allergies that have now suddenly appeared, with the bloating, gas and distension, or those alternating attacks of constipation and diarrhea, where should one start? An X-Ray of the bowels shows a "spastic colon", magic phrase for a symptomatic condition. Of course, medication does not help, and now, the patient becomes really concerned: she is gaining weight, she is constantly hungry and she has incredible cravings for sugar and other carbohydrates. Getting out of bed in the morning seems to be an impossible task, and if it were not for her cup of coffee, she would never make it to work. Depression and mood swings are the next step. "It is all in your head." "Go shopping." "Take a vacation." "Stop concentrating on your vagina and the discharge will go away." These are all well-meant pieces of "advice" from various doctors. Her family gets fed up with her "asocial" behavior and her chronic fatigue or "laziness."

The patient's relentless quest for the healer finally lands her on the couch of the psychiatrist. Her "vicious circle" is closed. Antidepressive medications cause severe "allergic" reactions and before she knows it, she finds herself in a psychiatric unit with a diagnosis of depression and sometimes even suicidal tendencies. Electric shocks and hospital food will do the rest. At this point, the patient may be convinced that she is suffering from at least an early Alzheimer. I feel great pity for Candida patients at this stage. Cut off from any support and subjected to hospital meals, they will get the final push over the brink to total depression. I wonder how many depressed patients we could find in those mental institutions that actually are Candida patients? We probably will never know.

One thing I know for certain: at least 75% of alcoholics do have a yeast problem. Have you ever wondered why recovering alcoholics go to their support groups (Alcoholics Anonymous meetings) for the rest of their lives? And why the alcohol addiction is swiftly replaced by a sugar addiction? Because the psychological support they get from their peers will not suppress the growth of the yeast cells, creating incredible cravings for carbohydrates. There is a physical dependency, which has to be corrected by a yeast-free diet, Lactobacilli supplements and yeast-killing drugs. Recovered alcoholics simply have replaced one addiction with another: alcohol with sugar. AA would do a great service to their members by explaining this in their lectures.

Another annoying symptom is the irritation and burning feeling of all the mucosae -- around the anus, the vagina, the mouth and the lips, and even the mucosae of the stomach -- which creates a constant feeling of hunger together with "cystitis" attacks, characterized by frequent, urgent and burning urination. Before he or she has a chance to think about it the patient is taking antibiotics, only to discover that many symptoms are aggravated. To the doctor's satisfaction, the patients' urine cultures are clear; but these "urinary infections" seem to come back with astonishing regularity. And they are accompanied by symptoms of "brain fog" as a result of which concentration and short-time memory are minimal. A Candida patient has to read everything at least three times more than anybody else, and to his or her despair, s/he is unable to retain it. Finally, the patient cannot balance their checkbook, or perhaps their work suffers to the degree that their boss thinks of dismissing them.

There are several symptoms that lead easily to a totally wrong therapy. We have already described the "cystitis" symptoms. Another frequent symptom is pressure in the ears, a fullness causing pain. This is common especially in children. Consequently, an "ear infection" is often diagnosed, although the real culprit is the yeast cell which causes retention of fluids. Swiftly, antibiotics are prescribed with catastrophic results, whereas inplantation of eartubes to drain the fluids would have been sufficient. I remember seeing an eighteen-month old girl, who was already on antibiotics for 14 months for recurrent "ear infections," with vaginal yeast. The child already manifested hyperactive behavior when eating sugar or chocolate.

Another annoying and frightening symptom of Candida is anxiety attacks, experienced even during therapy. They can be very severe, leading to a stay in the hospital, where doctors look in vain for the triggering factor. It is my observation that these anxiety attacks are caused by the accumulation of toxines, released by die-off. An enema or high doses of Vitamin C powder (1 tsp every hour) will clear these attacks.

Many symptoms are caused by the build-up of toxins, as already previously demonstrated. A very common, bizarre symptom is the metallic taste patients experience. It goes together with severe constipation and dry skin, all symptoms of toxicity and heat in the body. When those patients drink water, even the water tastes metallic. This frightening and unpleasant symptom disappears when there is a good evacuation of the toxins.

What is described above is not an exception, but rather the rule. Rejected by friends and family (because of ignorance or misunderstanding), Candida sufferers are angry and irritated, which isolates them even more from the love they need. Some want just to be left alone when they go through such a crisis, although they need, more than ever, a hug, someone to hold their hands or a sympathetic listener.

What makes things more complicated is that several immune-suppressed diseases have similar symptoms. CEBV and Candidiasis especially have several symptoms in common. And frighteningly, even ARC and AIDS patients have some of these same conditions. However, isn't this what we ought to expect? The root of the problem in all these conditions is a suppressed immune system; hence, the symptoms are those of a weak immune system, although in varying degree. Nevertheless, I have made an attempt, based upon my experience with the thousands of patients I have treated, to distinguish clinically CEBV from Candidiasis. This is reflected in Table # 6.

COMMON SYMPTOMS

1. "Brain fog": definite symptom in both conditions; difficulty concentrating, short-time memory disturbances, feeling of an early Alzheimer.

2. Irritability, drowsiness, blurred vision, pallor, cold extremities and extreme fatigue.

3. Insomnia, headaches, mood swings and depression.

4. Sensation of head swelling.

Table # 6

CEBV	CANDIDA
1. Intermittent attacks	1. Progressive, worsening course
2. No cravings for Carbo's / sugar	2. Irresistible cravings present
3. Very few gastrointestinal signs	3. Extreme constipation, gas, bloating, distension
4. No food sensitivities	4. Extreme food sensitivities, worsening with time
5. No skin rashes or nail infections	5. Skin rashes (butterfly rash on face) athlete's foot and nail infections often present
6. No postnasal drip	6. Postnasal drip constantly
7. No hormonal influence	7. Premenstrual worsening of symptoms, menstrual irregularities, amenorrhea
8. Muscle fatigue upon exertion	8. Muscle and joint pains most of the time

Table # 6 (continued)

CEBV	CANDIDA
9. No environmental sensitivities	9. Environmental sensitivities 60% of the time
10. No "cystisis" attacks	10. Recurrent "cystisis" attacks
11. No aggravation of symptoms in damp weather	11. Aggravation on damp, foggy days
12. No itching	12. Itching all over the body, anal and vaginal itching
13. Changes on tongue (redness, cracks) are on tip	13. Yellow, white fur in middle of tongue
14. No profuse perspiration	14. Profuse perspiration
15. No vaginal or urethral discharge	15. Vaginal and urethral discharge
16. No mucosal involvment	16. Mucosal involvement (trush, anal and vaginal)
17. Usually no anemia/ hypothyroidia present	17. Frequently anemia, hypothyroidy present
18. Chiropractic adjustments hold	18. Patient cannot hold chiropractic adjustment; one hour after adjustment patient is out of alignment again.

5. Weak, shaky muscles

6. Sore throats

7. Crying spells

8. Irritability

9. Chest congestion and palpitations

10. Feeling of being crazy or falling apart

11. Shortness of breath

12. Chills and low-grade fevers

13. Dizziness and light-headedness when standing up

14. Hypersensitivity towards sunlight and sound.

We always have to keep in mind that CEBV and Candidiasis go together in about 75% of the cases; these "mixed" infections make it difficult for the doctor to distinguish one condition from another. However, an experienced clinician will be able to make the differential diagnosis. And, of course, there are always the laboratory tests, discussed in paragraph D.

3. HOW DID WE ENCOURAGE THE GROWTH OF CANDIDA CELLS?

Of course, all the causes -- Hereditary Factors-Food-Emotions and External Factors -- leading to a depressed immune system can be responsible for an overgrowth of yeast cells (See Chapter One). However, there are some factors, standing out among the rest, which will inevitably lead to Candida.

The one group that predominates in the outbreak of Candida is the external group. When our first antibiotics became available during the Second World War (Penicillin), we had indisputably taken a big step forward; but things got somewhat out of hand after that initial period. Broad-spectrum antibiotics were -- and are -- used for common colds so that the normal flora (coli, bacteroides and enterobacteria) can be suppressed. We all know of the use of tetracyclines in the therapy of acne; low doses were, and still are, given for months at a time. In a few days, this results in a replacement of the normal flora with one that consists of resistant organisms, including the yeast. Ampicillin and Bactrim are frequently given for the wrong reasons, or because the public insist on strong medication for a cold, since it has no time (due to life's constraints) to heal more naturally. The "time-is-money" attitude which dictates this behavior is not necessarily the wisest long term approach, as we are discovering.

"I never took antibiotics in my life," some may say. Most likely they did, but didn't know it. Adding low doses of antibiotics to the feed of chickens, cows and pigs is routinely done. Although people who raise cows or pigs insist that they must use antibiotics to prevent infections and promote growth, knowledgeable critics are now "blowing the whistle" on them. The gravest threat is that regular feeding of antibiotics may produce resistant bacteria and lead to their multiplication in the flesh of animals. And here is the tragedy: this resistance to antibiotics is transferable to the person ingesting the meat of these animals.

Antibiotics are not the only "magic bullets" leading to yeast infections. Other factors are also well-recognized as creating opportunities for the conversion of Candida species from an innocent existence into a pathogen, invading all the tissues and organs. Cortisone preparations cause a fluctuation in the peripheral lymphocytes, exerting an immunosuppressive effect that increases the risk of candidiasis. Cytotoxic drugs used in cancer therapy cause a decrease in the white blood cells and will suppress the bone marrow, which is the production center of the body's defenders. The management of these patients allows organisms like Candida to invade the deep tissues. "The pill" -- sign of sexual liberation since 1952 -- creates other opportunities for Candida. The "pill" alters the vaginal secretions, elevating the glycogen content, which favors the growth of Candida. That Candida is influenced by hormonal disturbances is clearly seen in the third trimester of pregnancy and in the premenstrual period.

Hormonal fluctuations in the third trimester of pregnancy alter the vaginal secretions, elevating the glycogen content which again favors the growth of Candida. The progesterone increase before the menstrual cycle will increase the sugar content in the blood, enhancing the multiplication of yeast cells. No wonder women get these irresistible food cravings: no matter what they do, they seem to have no control over them.

As if this is not enough, other medical conditions favor the growth of Candida: burns, surgical interventions, indwelling catheters, hypothyroidism, ferriprive anemia and adult diabetes mellitus, conditions that have to be corrected in order to conquer the yeast completely.

4. HOW CAN WE ACCURATELY DIAGNOSE CANDIDA?

Above all, the clinical picture is the most important. Filling in a questionnaire and score sheet and mentioning triggering factors and symptoms will provide the patient with a good indication about possible yeast infections. The questionnaire is identical to the one outlined in Chapter One.

The next step is laboratory tests. Increased frequency of yeast isolations from sputum, urine, or feces should increase the index of suspicion in high-risk individuals. The most potentially useful yeast isolation, from the blood, has often proved unrewarding because of negative cultures in the presence of widespread infection. Of patients with invasive Candidiasis, up to 25% lack detectable antibodies to Candida; in other words, we will have a **negative** blood test in spite of the presence of the disease. Improvements in blood culture methods promise diagnostic gains.

Now I shall discuss the two most frequently used tests. The first is the Candida Antibody test. The principle of this test is that Candida, in normal circumstances, is present only in the gastrointestinal tract. The moment Candida cells arrive in the bloodstream, they are recognized as strange objects; hence, antibodies are formed. In the Candida Antibody test, three kinds of antibodies are measured: IgM, IgA and IgG. All of them must be below 100 MONA (Measure Of Normal Activity). Usually a patient with disseminated disease shows a figure of between 200 and 300. I have had patients with figures higher than 1,000. There are drawbacks to this test. Antibodies cannot be formed by the patient whose immune system is greatly suppressed (cancer and other far-advanced diseases); hence, normal levels can be found when the clinical picture is clearly positive. The second drawback is the waiting period of 14 days before the result is known.

The IgM antibody is the earliest formed antibody, peaking two weeks after exposure and disappearing fast. The IgG appears by the third day and will be the highest figure you get. However, if the person is chronically exposed, which is the case with with most Candida patients, only the IgA will give a response; there will be no IgG and IgM. The interpretation becomes highly subjective (See Fig.# 6). The Candida Antibody test is, in my experience, a lot less acurate, and I don't use it anymore in my practice.

The best and most accurate test available is the **CEIA** or **CandiSphere Enzyme Immuno Assay Test** (CERODEX LAB, Inc., P.O. Box 1151, Oklahoma City, OK. 73070), developed by immunologist David S. Bauman, Ph.D. This test is based on the fact that the Candida cell produces several molecules, which play a role in the production of symptoms. Some of these are alcohols, acetaldehyde and hormonal molecules (estrogen, progesterone, testosterone). These small molecules are directly responsible for the clinical effects of Systemic Candidiasis. Large molecules produced by Candida exert their effects directly and provide a mechanism for diagnosing the syndrome. One of these molecules is in the form of cytoplasmic proteins. They are the metabolic enzymes of Candida and are normally **not** found **outside** of the Candida cell. Hence, they are valuable to us as diagnostic probes. Normal figures are between 70 and 110. This is a big step forward in the diagnosis of Candida, since detection of any form of Candidiasis has historically been very difficult, because even "normal" individuals gave positive tests for antibodies.

Sometimes patients are puzzled as to why their laboratory figures go up in the first months, in spite of their feeling better. A similar phenomenon occurs with the antibody formation of the

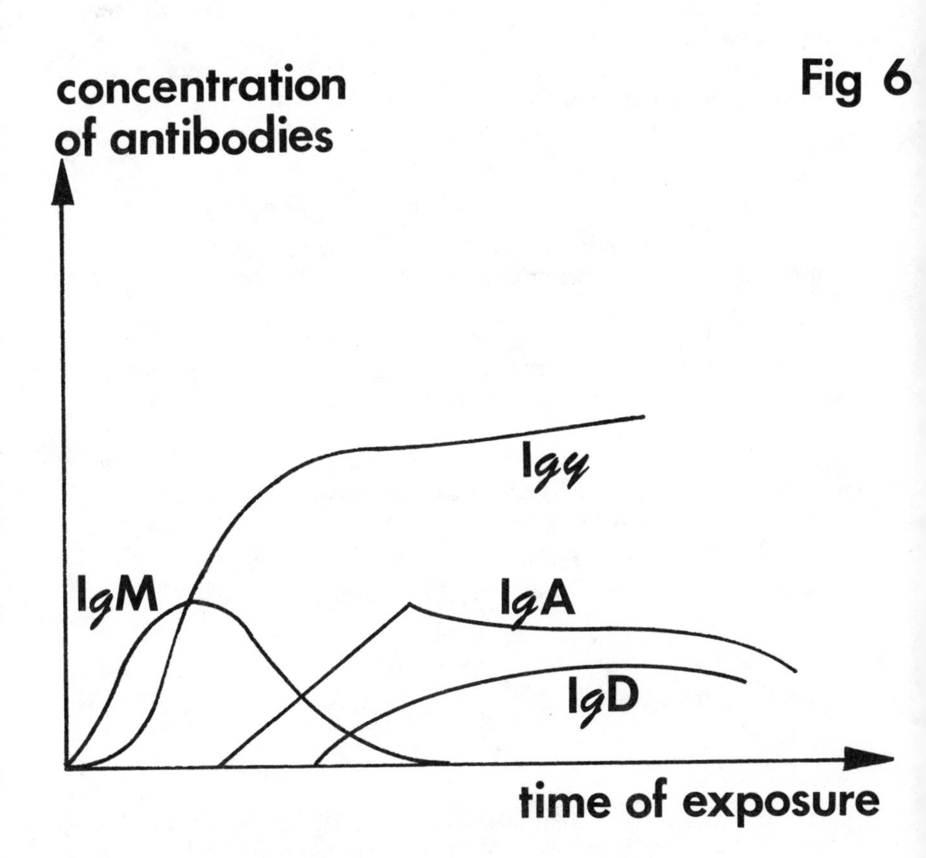

Candida Antibody Test

EBV. The figure below (Fig. # 7) indicates that with Nystatin therapy, the CEIA test will hit higher levels in the first three months, only to decrease markedly after six months to a year. What are the reasons for this? They can be twofold. First of all by killing Candida cells, you take away the immunosuppressive effect of the yeast cells from the immune system. Don't forget that this immune system is continually suppressed when you are exposed to a chronic Candida infection. By taking pressure away from the immune system, the latter is able to form more antibodies to fight the invaders, and only later, when the battle is won, do we see a decrease in the antibody formation.

Another factor to take into consideration is the **half-lifetime** of antibodies. The value is 21 days, after which length of time half of the original number amount of antibodies are still present.

A second reason for the initial increase in antibodies is the leaking of the proteins from disrupted Candida cells, thereby evoking an increase in antibody formation.

Another logical question would be: "Why do those antibodies that appear in CEBV and Candida not protect us from further infection?" The answer is because these antibodies do not kill. The killing is done by "natural killer cells" (NK cells), while antibodies are a reflection of the activity of our immune system.

In Table # 7, a comparason of diagnostic tests for chronic candidiasis is demonstrated.

5. THERAPY

The first and best treatment of any disease is the prevention of it. We have to pay close attention to all the triggering factors (as outlined in Chapter One). Of course, one that can be found in almost every patient is the overuse of antibiotics. We know that antibiotics are prescribed for nearly any infection, viral (where it will have no effect) and bacterial. Doctors and patients have become so used to antibiotics that they are frequently prescribed as a reflex. Often it takes all my eloquence to convince the patient not to take the antibiotic for a viral condition, since it is hazard-

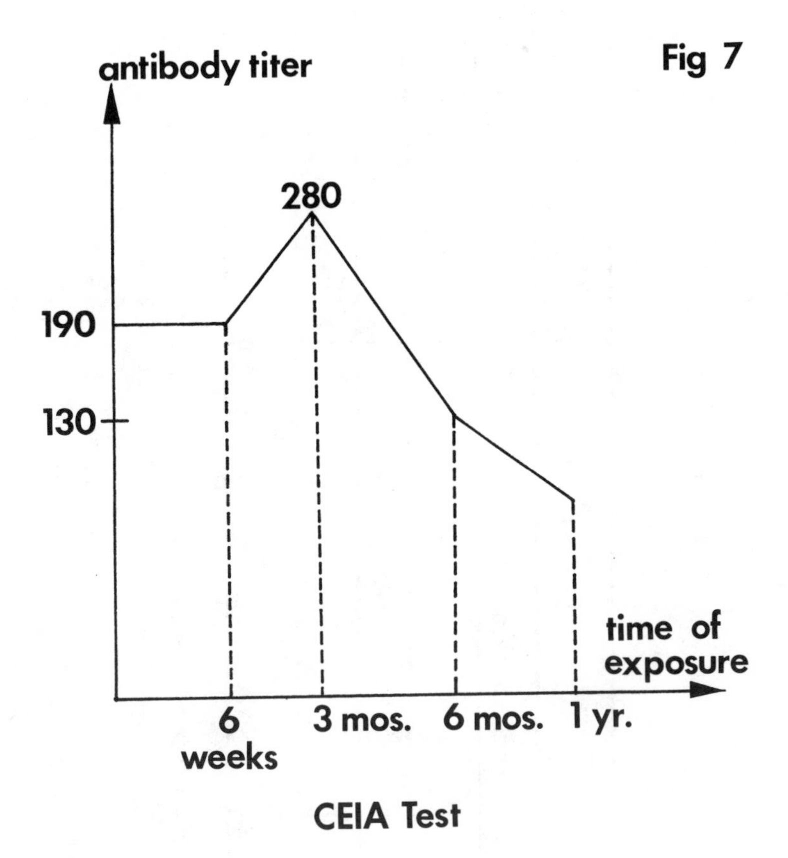

Fig 7

CEIA Test

Table # 7

	CEIA test	**Candida anti-body test**	**Skin test**
Detects what?	Antibodies against Candida proteins	Ab to Mannan	Cellular Immunity
Diagnostic test?	Yes	????	
Sensitivity	>88%	Unknown	N.A.
Specificity	>95%	Unknown	N.A.
Controlled study?	Yes	No	N.A.

Note: the Candida skin test is only useful when negative (it indicates immunosuppression); Mannan is part of the cell wall structure of Candida Albicans.

ous to his health. In almost all the medical histories of my patients, I notice the overuse of antibiotics. One of my very first question is, "When did you feel good for the last time and what happened?" Antibiotic intake is very frequently the triggering factor.

Of course, there are many indications for antibiotic intake. How do we protect ourselves then? By taking, from the start, a high daily dosage of Acidophilus (6 TBS of liquid) or Microflora (2 tbs daily in 2 oz. of water). It is such a pity that most doctors wait for the appearance of diarrhea before suggesting the intake of Acidophilus, and, at that, mostly in the form of yoghurt, which has a negligible concentration considering the purpose. Patients who are at that time on any antifungal medication should double their dosage for the duration of the antibiotic intake. Even for those patients who have not taken any medication, a maintenance dosage of an antifungal medication is advised.

Once we have taken care of the triggering factors (food, emotions, external factors), we are ready to start our battle against Candidiasis -- and a raging battle it is, requiring all the troops that we can muster. Here is the battle plan:

STARVE THE CANDIDA

KILL THE CANDIDA

REPLACE THE NORMAL FLORA

A. STARVE THE YEAST OR THE ANTI-YEAST DIET

Most of us "live to eat" instead of eating to live. Unfortunately, much of our social life is incorporated around food intake, which does not make it easier for a person to choose not to eat the regular diet. But eating properly for your particular needs is simply a common-sense way of life. Certainly hunger has little to do with many of our eating patterns, but this most of us have yet to learn. I remember as a child my grandfather giving me candy as a daily treat. When I ended up getting sick, the amount of "goodies" was even increased; grandpa did not know that the excess sugar was responsible for my troubles in the first place.

So often we adults are trying to fill an emotional void, and it becomes a bottomless pit. We sit down to eat and do not want to stop. The purpose of "shoveling the food in" is to fill that bottomless emotional hole which, of course, can never be filled by eating. Oddly enough, although this may have been a lifetime habit, we only seem to become aware of it when we make changes in our diet.

If we know that Candida cells are such voracious eaters, consuming almost anything for their growth, we had better pay attention to their favorite foods, **carbohydrates** (especially sugars) and **fermented** foods! So let's stop these pointless questions: "When can I stop this boring diet?" "When can I add sugar?" "When can I have some wine or alcoholic drinks?"

Fortunately for most patients, we can return in moderation to most of the foods after 2 months. I said foods, not "junk food." What is encouraging to see is that most patients feel so revived with their new diet, it becomes their "normal" diet -- a "jewel on their crown" of health for the rest of their lives. Your willingness to improve the quality of your life through more healthful food choices and meal planning is a very significant step toward better health, and your efforts will produce the desired result. Following a healthful diet will make you more aware of the "garbage" that people eat. You will be motivated to do better and acquire. the energy, the body, health, mental and physical powers, that you always dreamed of. Let's look at the list of forbidden and allowed foods.

FORBIDDEN FOODS

- Breads: including yeast-free wheat and rye breads. However, rice and corn breads, unleved and ponce breads are O.K.

- Dairy products: except butter, eggs and goat's milk, goat's cheese and yoghurt; other yoghurt is not allowed.

- Mushrooms, wine, champagne and beer or anything else that is fermented, such as Miso and tofu.

- Fruits: especially not apples, pears and grapes; also no watermelon, cantaloupe, oranges, peaches, prunes, dates or dried fruits (too much sugar).

- Wheat and Rye: in crackers, cereal, breads and pasta.

- Avoid salt: prefer sea salt if used. Absolutely **no sugar** in any form; avoid Aspartame (Nutrasweet, Sweet-N-Low), no honey, molasses or maple syrup.

- No tea or coffee, not even caffeine-free coffee, or herbal teas; exceptions are mentioned further. No fruit juices except the juices of allowed fruits; even then, use them sparingly; and certainly do NOT use fruit juices when fasting.

- No tomato or barbecue sauce (unless you make your own without peppers, sugar, vinegar, syrup).

- Avoid raw and cold foods (except salads **occasionally**; more about salads is discussed further). Remember, these foods decrease the strength of your digestive organ, the spleen-pancreas as outlined in Chapter One.

- Absolutely no vinegar: in salad dressings, mustard and mayonnaise.

- No oatmeal, horseradish, peppers.

- No canned foods or fried foods.

- Avoid refrigerated left-overs, especially meat; freeze the left-overs and heat them up later (this is especially the rule for meats, since they will become damp and moldy overnight).

- Avoid ice in drinks.

ALLOWED FOODS

- Water with lemon juice.

- Vegetable juices freshly sqeezed (**not** canned such as V8).

- Cranberry juice (unsweetened).

- Wheatgrass juice.

- Fruit juices of allowed fruits (in moderation).

- Goat's milk.

- Coconut milk

- Papaya, mango, kiwi, pineapple, banana, honeydew melon, coconut, guava and lemons. A word of caution here: use fruits only in the morning, for breakfast; do not eat after other meals. Some people (10%) will not be able to eat fruit at all because of the high fructose content or acidity (banana, pine-apple).

- Chicken, turkey, lamb, veal and rabbit.

- Most fish, preferably cold-water fish (salmon, true cod, sea bass); avoid trout and orange roughy.

- All vegetables, steamed, cooked or stir-fried; avoid eating them raw.

- Lettuce with tomatos, avocados, and lemon with linseed or avocado oil as salad dressing.

- Butter and eggs.

- Nuts (except peanuts and pistachios) and seeds, nut butter (except peanut butter).

- Rice cakes, rice crackers, corn tortillas, corn chips, "Rice and Shine."

- Quinoa, amaranth, buckwheat, millet, wild rice, brown rice; avoid white rice, it has no nutritional value.

- Corn, popcorn.

- Beans.

- Rice noodles and Japanese buckwheat noodles.

- Goat's cheese and goat's yoghurt.

Do we improve **immediately** on this diet? Not exactly. The area of greatest misunderstanding and confusion in the field of nutrition is the failure to properly understand and interpret the changes and symptoms that follow the beginning of an improved nutritional program. When we introduce foods of higher quality in place of lower-quality ones, we have to understand the sudden onset of new, and not-always-improved, symptoms. This is exactly what happens to the Candida patient when s/he switches from junk food or food rich in yeast to a protein-rich quality diet. A cleansing process has to take place, which requires enormous amounts of energy, giving the patient a feeling of exhaustion and heaviness. And considering the years we have abused our bodies, our clean-up operation will not be done in a couple of days, but rather will require a couple of weeks or months. The quality of a nutritional program is also improved by omitting toxic substances such as coffee, tea, chocolate, frozen yoghurt, salt, tobacco, etc.

A few important rules have to be remembered by the patient who wants to recover from illness through a high-quality diet. There is no doubt: the **higher** the quality of food we eat, the **quicker** we recover from disease, provided, of course, we are able to properly digest and assimilate.

Should following these rules give us joy, a state of well-being and relaxation? Not quite; at least not immediately. The body still has to discard lower-grade materials and make room for these improved superior replacements. Many patients fall into the trap of stopping their new diet in this phase. "I feel better on the junk diet -- the new one makes me feel weak."

Of course, initially and usually between the third and tenth day of the diet, we experience "**die-off symptoms.**" Due to the formation of toxins, the die-off symptoms can be any of the Candida symptoms, even in exacerbated form. These symptoms classically start around the second day of treatment and can last as long as two weeks, and in extreme cases even longer, up to months. However, because yeast cells are not discriminating in their food choice (they can consume almost anything for their growth, including mucus), even following the diet faithfully will not always avoid die-off. Among the symptoms some stand out:

. Headaches.

. Muscle-and-joint pains; the patient feels flu-like symptoms or symptoms that resemble an acute arthritis attack.

. Running nose, formation of mucus in the sinuses, imitating "sinusitis" or coughing up of a greenish, yellow sputum.

. Mucus in greenish stools.

. Vaginal discharge: cheesy, white discharge, imitating the vaginal Candida infection; however, culture for yeast is negative.

. "Cystitis" symptoms: frequent, urgent and painful urination; culture of the urine is negative.

. Sudden brain fog, feeling of being drunk.

The course of these symptoms is characteristic a fluctuating pattern, with symptoms being present at a given time, then disappearing two hours later and finally reappearing many hours later. This "roller-coaster" phenomenon is due to the presence of toxins. When the gastrointestinal tract is relatively free of toxins, patients feel relatively good; two hours later the toxin build-up will overwhelm the patients. Their sudden changes in behavior that results does not always contribute to the acceptance of the disease by friends or family members.

HOW DO WE AVOID OR ALLEVIATE THE DIE-OFF SYMPTOMS?

Follow the anti-yeast diet as strictly as possible, especially during the first three to four weeks; each time you cheat, you give the yeast cells a chance to grow, prolonging the period of die-off.

Be sure to stay with your medication intake; it does not help very much when you forget your medication half of the time; a medication sitting on your shelf does not work!

Probably the best self-help for the die-off is the assurance of a good bowel movement; at least once a day the patient has to move his bowels or toxins will build up to an intolerable level. Many natural laxatives are available, one of the best being "Colonic Rinse", by Vitality Products (818-889-7739). Other excellent products are Perfect Seven, Swiss Kriss Tea, Super Dieters Laci Lebeau Tea, flaxseeds, senna seeds -- all available in your local health food store. Avoid psyllium seeds, they will rather constipate. Psyllium will be more indicated in case of loose bowel movements, alternated with constipation, but ask for the psyllium husk. If necessary, an enema should be taken. Again, during the first three weeks, everything should be done to ensure this evacuation.

Change your diet to a high-fiber one: increase it by the amount of **allowed** fruits, vegetables, nuts, rice bran and brown rice that you serve. An extremely good product for evacuation of toxins is Celginate (General Research Laboratories or GRL, 818-349-9911. The tablet contains sea algae combined with celery root powder, making it an excellent bulking agent. It improves the bowel movement; the algae absorb many of the toxins; therefore, consumption of this product helps clear the skin. Start with a dose of three tablets with each meal; you may increase to five, three times a day.

For the vaginal "yeast" discharge, douche with lactobacillus liquid (GRL), dissolved in either three TBS of water or two TBS of plain yoghurt. You can add to this "cocktail" one TBS of liquid garlic and 1 TBS of Pau D'Arco tea. Douche for a week, every evening.

For the "cystitis" symptoms, take unsweetened cranberry juice (dilute it half and half with water) or, when the burning is too severe, ask your doctor to add Pyridium 200 mg, one tablet three times a day. Avoid acidic foods: beef and pork, pineapple, tomato, and other irritating substances, such as coffee, tea, and tobacco smoke. If this does not help, and a true cystitis is excluded through a urine culture, add 1/8 tsp of Nystatin powder twice a day, mixed in some water. It is one of the very few excellent medical indications of Nystatin remaining.

In spite of the above measures, a lot of patients keep on experiencing extreme constipation, excessive bloating and heavy brain fog. I would do a disfavor to my readers if I did not mention **the** therapy to resolve these unpleasant effects: **Colonic Hydrotherapy.** Excessive toxin formation will block regular elimination, thereby making the passage of waste material entirely too slow. The colon loses its ability to have regular peristaltic action, nerve signals stop functioning and the feces gradually lodge in pockets. Dehydration or drying out of the stool takes place. This toxic debris is gradually reabsorbed via the blood back into the system, creating toxemia. These problems can be remedied by colonic hydrotherapy while avoiding dependency on habit forming laxatives.

Generally the more laxatives one takes the more one needs to increase the dose to stimulate the colon. Four hundred million dollars are spent annually on laxatives in the United States. The use of laxatives creates dehydration in the body; many layers of dried feces remain in the colon because with laxatives only more recent feces are pushed through the center and evacuated. With colonic therapy, the gentle cleansing and regeneration of the colon can begin. The first recorded use of colon hydrotherapy was in 1500 B.C., when it was described as the infusion of aqueous substance into the large intestine through the anus. Today, with modern technological advances, safe, effective, and sterile instrumentation is available for this healthy modality of the past. Using gentle infusion with pressure-controlled, purified water, the treatment is designed to cleanse all the way through to the cecum at the beginning of the colon.

The individual lies on his or her back and the trained operator gently inserts a small disposable tube in the anus. The gentle purified water is mechanically infused in and out of the colon without assistance from the individual. The outflow of water removes excess gas, mucus, feces and infectious material. During the entire cycle, the operator may gently massage the abdomen to loosen gas and feces from the colon. Guided by an experienced therapist, there is no danger of dependency, while the cleaner colon makes the process of elimination easier and overall health is enhanced. I do not hesitate to say: boosting of your immune system starts with the cleansing of your colon.

WHAT DO WE DO WITH THESE CRAVINGS FOR SWEETS AND OTHER CARBOHYDRATES?

Anyone who suffers from Candidiasis knows that cravings can rule their life. There is an irresistible urge, a driven feeling for the body to consume certain foods. It can turn people into nervous wrecks, into irritable, angry tyrants who lose control over their actions and thinking. What do these cravings mean -- do they fulfill certain basic physiological needs? Let's see first what modern medicine thinks about this.

My attention was drawn to the inadequacies of the Western explanation of "cravings" when I was visiting a friend in Boston and he handed me the "Good Health Magazine", part of the **New York Times Magazine**, which contained an article, entitled: "Does Your Body Know What It Needs? Cravings." Reading this article I was astonished at the very poor explanation by various eminent researchers. Different opinions ranged as follows: "There is no physiological reason to explain these cravings." (Dr. Richard Mattes, Monell Chemical Center in Philadelphia). "These foods are craved because their consumption will either satisfy a nutritional deficiency or, particularly with carbohydrate cravings (attention Candida-sufferers!), serve as a form of self-medication to counteract depression." Whoever says this has never witnessed the deep depressions or suicidal tendencies of Candida patients after consuming these foods.

Other opinions included the following: "carbohydrate cravings are linked to people with seasonal depressions, and therefore, what they crave is actually what they need." (Dr. Norman Rosenthal, psychiatrist at the National Institute of Mental Health). It is a fact that women report cravings more often than men, most likely because of food desires related to menstruation and pregnancy, according to Dr. Harvey Anderson, Chairman of the Department of Nutritional Sciences at the University of Toronto Medical School. He found that carbohydrate consumption increases by 30% just prior to menstruation.

Another study at Kansas State University by Katharina Grunewald, Associate Professor of Foods and Nutrition, found that most of these women craved chocolate more during menstruation than at any other time of the month. Cravings for popcorn, potato chips and hamburgers were not increased by the menstrual cycle. She states: "We don't know why women crave more chocolate during the menstrual cycle, we simply know they do. It may be that they want to do something pleasant for themselves."

To me it seems that modern medicine has more questions than answers on the issue of food cravings. We already briefly mentioned the influence of taste as it was known in Chinese medicine (Page 22). Is it possible that acupuncture knows the answers to the above questions and, in fact, has known them for more than 50 centuries?

The Chinese knew that when you craved a certain food, and in reality we need to say a certain taste, the organ belonging to the taste was suffering (See Fig. # 3). The spleen-pancreas is suffering when we crave sweets and other carbohydrates (CBH). So to some extent it is true that their consumption will satisfy a nutritional deficiency: the **moderate** consumption of CBH (if at all possible -- extreme cases of Candida will not tolerate this at all) and sweets will strengthen the spleen-pancreas. However, when patients experience cravings, we usually do not think in terms of "moderate amounts." Usually the patient can get on a roller coaster of sugar intake, having quite the opposite effect of what we are discussing. The high amount of sweetness will knock down the energy in the spleen-pancreas. As I have seen in my practice with Candida sufferers (and we are talking here about millions of individuals), consumption of sugar or CBH will improve their mood for only a very short time (half an hour). Afterwards, inevitably, they will collapse with severe mood swings and depression, sometimes suicidal tendencies. As Traditional Chinese Medicine shows, it is a very fine balance of intake of sweet taste, different from individual to individual, that will balance the deficient organ, or as we express it in modern medicine, that will satisfy the nutritional deficiency.

Every woman with Candida will have PMS and experience severe cravings for CBH, especially sweets. In fact, we often see that even when patients with Candida get rid of their cravings for the rest of the month, the week before the menstrual bleeding spells bad news for sweets eaters. The answer is simple. The progesterone increase before the menstrual cycle leads to an increased glycemia (sugar) in the blood. This is music to the ears of the yeast cell, which starts multiplying faster, sensing the presence of increased sugar. So it is simply the **yeast cells'** cravings; they want you to feel their cravings and most patients oblige. What a disaster for these patients to follow the advice of Dr. Rosenthal, who claims that what they crave is actually what they need! Millions of Candida sufferers will refute this: increased sugar intake would lead them, more probably, to the brink of suicide.

HOW CAN WE COPE WITH THESE CRAVINGS?

We certainly don't surrender. It is wonderful to see how cravings disappear when we omit the very foods that we crave. Contrary to the consensus of the medical experts quoted in the NY Times, I would say that cravings are alarm signals to warn the patient to eliminate the food or taste that is craved. Easier said than done, you say. Well, there is some help available. Acupuncture has certain points that can cut the cravings immediately, even before the adjustment to the diet is made. We also have **Carnithine**, an amino acid that can cut cravings (2-3 tablets daily). This is usually sufficient to get the patient over the initial craving. Also GTF Chromium, which will regulate the sugar-insulin balance, can be very helpful if taken twice a day. Another excellent product is Green Magma, 6 tablets a day before meals. Even if patients are tempted by some sweets, many are surprised to discover that these sweets no longer taste "as good as they used to.

YOU CAN SELECT FOODS TO INCREASE YOUR ENERGY AND AVOID THE MOOD SWINGS!

This is music to the ears of all immuno-suppressed patients. But in fact, you can manage the food you eat to alleviate disturbing symptoms such as insomnia, morning fatigue as well as the inevitable depressions and mood swings. As you can imagine, not all foods will be able to give you these quick positive changes in mood. As explained earlier, the Candida diet is a high-protein, low-carbohydrate one. This is just what the doctor ordered for your symptoms.

For most people, protein will increase the morning vigor, avoid the post-lunch doldrums and keep one's energy up throughout the day. Of course, not all protein will have the same effect. The most effective energy boosters will be the proteins low in fat: fish, shellfish, veal, chicken without the skin and **very** lean beef. For healthy people not suffering from Candida, low-fat milk and low-fat yoghurt will have the same effect.

On the other hand, if you want to achieve a calming and more relaxing effect, one that will reduce anxiety and let you fall asleep more readily, carbohydrates are in order. There are two types: the sugars (glucose, sucrose, fructose and lactose) or the starchy carbohydrates (potatoes, corn, and vegetables).

The conclusion is simple: eating more protein will boost **your energy**, eating more carbohydrates will calm you down and sometimes make you sleepy. How come? Small chunks of information are transported from one brain cell to another by means of chemical substances, called **neurotransmitters**. There are two classes of these chemicals manufactured by the brain from the foods we eat: the "alertness" chemicals (Dopamine and Norepinephrine) and the "calming" chemical, Serotonin. The precursor or aminoacid of the Dopamine and Norepinephrine is **Thyrosine**, the precursor of the serotonin is **Tryptophan**. These two amino acids will enter the brain with other essential amino acids. They will try to gain access to the brain through the **Brain-Blood**

Barrier. Let's visualize this.

Your group of amino acids are sitting on an airfield strip, maneuvering with each other to gain access to the take-off area. However, Tryptophan is the least plentiful amino acid in the blood. So you have one "airplane" of Tryptophan, surrounded by many other "airplanes" of competing amino acids. It gets worse when you eat more protein: so many other "airplanes" will sit on those side strips that you actually can **deplete** your Tryptophan. So what's the solution? That's easy -- eat more carbohydrates in the evening when you want the calming effect of serotonin to fall asleep (important when we know that insomnia is a constant symptom of Candida sufferers).

Besides regulating the glucose balance, insulin has yet another important function: it will keep those amino acids moving in the bloodstream to join up with our cells. However, Tryptophan tends to be "anchored" to albumin in the blood and finds itself all of a sudden in a favorable position to get past the blood-brain barrier through lack of competition. Candida sufferers should get the protein in their breakfast and lunch when they need energy. They should eat their CBHs at night with little protein, to ensure a calming effect.

Do we need supplemental Tryptophan and Thyrosine? Most Candida patients do. They often have a malabsorption problem, thus less of those amino acids will arrive in the bloodstream. Take Thyrosine 1000 mgs (GRL), one in the morning, one in the afternoon and a 600 mg capsule Tryptophan (GRL), 1/2 hour before going to bed.

Clearly it is **not** a matter of luck to feel energetic and happy. Applying the above information can modify your moods and assure you effectiveness and motivation in helping yourself fight your suppressed immune system.

A WORD ABOUT OUR SALADS

There are chocolate-lovers and salad addicts. Addicts, I hear you say? Aren't salads going to make me slender and beautiful? A minimum of calories, lots of roughage to ensure bowel movement – a nutritional dream. Not quite. Salad, an attractive vegetable for fungi, insects and birds, has developed a whole arsenal of weapons against these enemies. Alas, one defense mechanism will rob the fanatic salad eater from his or her one possible excuse: that salads are nutritional. Salads have "nutritional blockers," products that will bind with vitamins, preventing their absorption. For instance, oxalic acid in spinach blocks the absorption of calcium and iron, not necessarily what you want in a Candida-diet, where calcium intake is already low.

Another unwanted effect of some raw vegetables (such as bamboo sprouts, cashews and peanuts), is the presence of protease inhibitors: they hamper the action of the protein enzymes.

Even more important to all patients suffering from an overload of toxins (as is the case with Candida) salad ingredients manufacture these poisons, especially the ones that have been attacked by fungi and insects. Examples are lima beans, unripe millet and bamboo shoots. The toxins present are destroyed by proper cooking. The list is endless, but virtually ignored. But the message is clear: don't eat salads every day. Vitamin blockers, toxins and artificial food additives and coloring substances, make our salads less desirable than they seem.

B. KILL THE CANDIDA

After being abused by medications for so long, most patients are not very enthusiastic about returning to any medication. This is understandable. However, Candida is a tough enemy. It took clever advantage of your weakened immune system in order to invade your body. Once inside, the yeast cells continue to suppress your defense mechanism. This is where the anti-yeast medication plays a very important role in breaking the vicious circle. Compare this to an attack on your enemy defending his position in his castle. You could opt for starving him out by cutting off his food-supply lines, or you could both starve him and attack his fortress. It is clear that the second option, although a tough one, is the most effective. Choosing the best weapons is the most important step. There are two types: natural products and medications.

1. NATURAL PRODUCTS

a. Garlic

Garlic has a long history of medicinal use. It dates back to the Babylonians, the Pharaohs and the Greeks. Louis Pasteur, the famous microbiologist, and more recently, Albert Schweitzer, were firm believers in garlic for its antimicrobial and antibacterial activity. Garlic is a natural antifungal, extremely helpful for all Candida patients. It is often the **only** thing that relieves bloating and gas. It lessens the intestinal pain and burning often experienced. Fresh garlic in salads also relieves water retention in the body. If you can't take digestive enzymes, garlic will help in digesting the food. As you can see, garlic is extremely helpful and important in the anti-Candida regimen. Take at least two TBS of liquid garlic mixed in water or allowed juice, or at least six deodorized capsules with meals. When we add that garlic has been proven to be effective in lowering the cholesterol, then we have a sure winner on our hands.

b. H2O2, Dioxychlor and Aerox

The relief of tissue hypoxia (lack of oxygen) has been the subject of many investigative studies. Early investigators infused oxygen intravenously with limited success. As far back as 1904, dying tuberculose patients were treated with intravenous oxygen. The patients' pulse and respiration improved, but for unknown reasons, the treatment was not repeated and the patients died.

In 1916 intravenous oxygen diminished the cyanosis (blue color of lips and cheeks) of critically ill patients. The first use of Hydrogen Peroxide (H2O2) was reported in 1920, in patients with Influenzal Pneumonia. By using Hydrogen Peroxide the mortality rate of those patients was markedly reduced.

In modern days intravenous infusions of H2O2 have been given without serious side-effects. Acutely ill patients with infection, allergy reactions, flu syndromes and other toxic phenomena had rapid improvement with infusion of H2O2. Food-grade H2O2 has been used with excellent results in the fight against Candida. It is taken either orally, 1 TBS twice a day, or intravenously in a saline solution.

Dioxychlor and Aerox are the next generation of oxygen suppliers. They are inorganic oxidants, useful against three major classes of infective agents -- viruses, bacteria and fungi. Perhaps the biggest contribution of Dioxychlor might be in the battle against environmental disease -- particularly the multiple-sensitivity condition, generally denominated "Universal Reactor Syndrome" (URS). This syndrome is almost always characterized by Systemic Candidiasis and multiple allergies and sensitivities. The Universal Reactor Syndrome is a situation in which the patient increasingly becomes sensitive to virtually everything in the environment. Patients react to things ranging from actual industrial chemicals to simple foods, even to the clothing they wear or the sheets they sleep on. URS becomes a traumatic daily struggle in which an already depressed immune system is constantly turning against itself. It leads to unrelenting daily torture.

H2O2 is available here in the United States in homeopathic drops, but it is administered intravenously in Mexico.

c. Pau d'Arco

Quickly gaining popularity is the South American herb Pau d'Arco, which is often refered to by its other Spanish names: Ipe Roxa, Lapacho and Taheebo. It is currently hailed for its effects on abdominal cancer (in South America) and Candida. Pau D'Arco is the inner bark of a large tree that flowers in a vibrant pink, purple or yellow, depending on the species. Throughout South America Pau D'Arco is used as a remedy for immune system-related problems, such as colds, fevers, infections and snake bites, but even more important for us, the bark has natural anti-fungal properties. It was one of the major healing herbs used by the Incas. The toxicity of Pau D'Arco is very low. It may loosen the bowels, which is frequently desirable in the Candida patient. It is available in capsules and tea bags.

2. ANTIFUNGAL DRUGS AND SUPPLEMENTS

a. Nystatin Powder

Nystatin powder was the initial drug of choice in treating the Candida patient. However, at this point it is totally outdated -- and for very good reasons. First of all, it is rather expensive and very few pharmacies carry it. A major disadvantage is that Nystatin is **not** a broad-spectrum fungicide. While effective for certain strains of Candida, numerous potentially pathogenic fungi are unaffected by it. With prolonged use, it leads to the development of resistance to the drug and continued symptoms. Nystatin is a mold by-product and may cause allergic reactions in the mold-sensitive patient.

Some adverse reactions are nausea and vomiting, while withdrawal symptoms are usually noted when the Nystatin is halted. This is not unusual, as I have seen patients who were on Nystatin for several years! In the generic sense, Nystatin is a potent antibiotic and the long-term effects of its use on normal bacterial and normal fungal intestinal flora are not clear. It is obvious from the above facts that if your doctor prescribes Nystatin for Systemic Candidiasis, it is time to look for another doctor. It can be used locally, such as for vaginal discharge and itching, or it can be sniffed for the postnasal drip. As previously mentioned, still a major indication of Nystatin powder is to counteract the frequent painful urination the patient experiences at night and during the day. You can start with 1/8 of a tsp building it up to 1/2 tsp twice a day.

b. Nizarol tablets, 200 mg (Ketoconazole)

This is a very potent antifungal drug. It is a synthetic broad-spectrum antifungal agent available in white tablets, each containing 200 mg ketoconazole.

In my opinion, it is not a first-line drug for Systemic Candidiasis since adverse reactions such as nausea and vomiting and, more disturbing, liver damage can occur. A blood test before and after use of it is mandatory. It is easy to take, since only one tablet daily is required. I like to prescribe it after my initial 5-week treatment with my first-choice supplements, especially in cases where the Candida is present mainly in the esophagus, ear, nose or throat.

c. Capryllin (GRL)

Scientific literature has long indicated that Caprylic acid should be effective in killing Candida Albicans. Capryllin (GRL) responded to that demand effectively. It is formulated as a time-release preparation. The coating of Capryllin allows for slow release of Caprylic acid along the entire length of the gastro-intestinal tract. Start with **one** capsule with meals, three times a day for the first two days. Increase to two tablets, three times a day, for the next three days. Continue with three tablets, three times a day, for the next five days and finish with four capsules, three times a day, for two weeks. Then, go to a maintenance dosage of two tablets twice a day for one month at least, after which time each patient must be evaluated individually. **Always** take Capryllin with meals, since it is an acid and as such can cause stomach pain and gastritis. It is not unusual that the maintenance dosage has to be continued for at least three months.

d. Homeopathic Herbal products

This is the most revolutionary and effective method I have encountered for the thousands of patients I have treated. This method is the future therapy, the most efficient and extremely fast-working. It is discussed in Chapter eight.

C. REPLACE THE NORMAL FLORA

The normal intestinal flora comprises three parts. The main flora consists of Anaeroba bacteria (Bacterium Bifidus and Bacteroides). The secondary flora is composed of the E. Coli, Enterococci and Lactobacilli. The third contains Yeast Cells, Clostridia and Staphylococci. We already know that the presence of these billions of friendly bacteria (L. Acidophilus and Bifidobacterias) are essential in order to inhibit the growth of yeast cells. Normal flora can be destroyed after only a few days with antibiotics and need to be replaced in order to avoid the creation of a favorable environment for the yeast. By supplementing your daily diet with stable, high potency L. Acidophilus and Bifidobacteria, you are greatly enhancing your body's natural ability to keep dangerous and/or pathogenic micro-organisms under control.

There are many people who would benefit greatly from using L. Acidophilus supplements, but who feel that they cannot successfully do so due to lactose intolerance or other milk-based allergies. They reluctantly purchase so-called "hypo-allergenic" or "milk-free" products that claim to be superior in potency and viability due to the absence of milk in their processing methods. However, what the public is not aware of is the fact that by not culturing their microorganisms in a milk base, the viability and potency are severely impaired.

Also it is known that lactose-intolerant patients do not manufacture "lactase," which is a naturally occurring enzyme whose function it is to break down milk sugar into a more simple form which the body can then digest. However, by introducing very small amounts of a high-quality acidophilus product into the system on a daily basis over an extended period of time, the natural production of lactase will be stimulated, and the body will begin to take care of this function on its own. Therefore, the optimum way to conquer milk-based allergies is to introduce various strains of acidophilus bacteria into the system in small increments (1/16-1/8 tsp once daily) and gradually increase these amounts weekly to the minimum recommended dosage of 1/2 tsp daily.

Looking at all the brands available on the market, it might be very difficult for the consumer to make a choice. From my experience one of the best products available is Lactobacillus liquid and Lactobacillus capsules from GRL. The normal dosage of the liquid is 1 tbs after each meal, or one capsule after each meal. This product is also excellent for vaginal yeast infections -- douche with 1 tbs Lactobacillus in 3 ounces of water for several evenings. As its taste is close to that of yoghurt, it is the preferred and favorite acidophilus preparation to give your children in case of constipation or other gastrointestinal disturbances.

However, don't fall into the trap of purchasing cheap, fruit-flavored acidophilus brands. They are far inferior to the above product and are a waste of money. Another important fact is that once you open a bottle of acidophilus (powder, capsules or liquid), you must keep it in the refrigerator to preserve the quality of the viable microorganisms in it.

In spite of using the above products in my practice for quite some time, I sensed that there was a shortcoming in the restoration of the normal flora. , And one of the most important steps in the therapy of Candida and any other immuno-suppressed condition is the restoration of a flora as close as possible to nature. Failure to do so will inevitably lead to to relapses of Candida, no matter what medications are taken to kill these yeast cells. Sofar, the products on the market, mainly the Lactobacillus products, sometimes mixed with Bifido bacteria and Bulgaricus, are given with mixed result.

My attention was brought to another new product on the market, **Microflora or Superflora**. Working with the product I was excited about the results. Microflora is a more complete system for helping the body to restore bacterial balance. It has many more advantages. Its price is lower than the available Acidophilus products. It is suitable for people with Lactose intolerance, which is no small deal considering the amount of Candida sufferers, having a Lactase deficiency. It does not require refrigeration, it is stored at room temperature, which makes it easier to travel. **All** Acidophilus products on the other side, require refrigeration. And the shelf life time is six months, considerably longer than the Acidophilus.

Who should take Microflora (Superflora)?

It is a must in immuno-suppressed conditions such as Candida, Chronic Epstein Barr Virus, and other Herpes Simples viruses. It should be taken as a **reflex** when antibiotics are administered, orally or intravenously in order to avoid overgrowth of yeast and reactivation of latent viruses. Gastrointestinal disorders such as gastritis, stomach-and duodenal ulcers, Colitis Ulcerosa and Crohn's disease will benefit from a restoration of the normal intestinal flora. In fact looking at the causes of immuno-suppressed conditions, this product can be taken as a **preventive** measure by everyone, children included. Anyone taking Acidophilus should replace it with Microflora (Superflora).

What is the dosage?

- Adults should mix 2 tbs of Microflora with 2 ounces of water. Take at least 15 minutes before eating.

- Children age 2 to 6 years of age, should take 1 tbs added to 1 ounce of water.

To obtain this product, write or phone to:

Micro-Flora Corporation,
Old Conejo Road # 115
Newbury Park, CA 91320
Tel: (805) 499-0615

6. DIFFERENTIAL DIAGNOSIS

Due to the generality of the symptoms and the lack of adequate laboratory tests, doctors have a tendency to focus on certain symptoms of the patient in particular. Therefore, certain devastatingly inaccurate diagnoses are made, devastating because they indicate incurable diseases. Whenever I see patients in my practice or during a speaking engagement, I meet unfortunate souls who were diagnosed with one of the following three conditions: M.S. or Multiple Sclerosis; S.L.E. or Systemic Lupus Erythomatosis; and Interstitial Cystitis. Unfortunately, there are plenty of people out there suffering from one of these conditions. However, it would be wise for the doctor and the patient to first rule out the diagnosis of Candida. Even if the diagnosis of these autoimmune diseases is confirmed, the patients can greatly benefit from the Candida diet. Let's have a closer look at these three conditions.

a. Multiple Sclerosis.

This condition hits at a young age, especially females between 30 and 45 years old. The disease may take one of two forms: either a relapsing, remitting disease of the nervous system (there is a degeneration of the myelin sheet around the nerves) or a chronic progressive disease. Symptoms can be double vision, incontinence, fatigue, dizziness, and numbness and weakness in an extremity. The latter symptoms might be confused with Candida. We have to keep in mind that there is not one single test that indicates with 100% certainty that one suffers from M.S. Rather a battery of tests is done: spinal tap, evoked potentials and NMR

(Nuclear Magnetic Resonance) to show possible demyelinating plaques in the brain or spinal cord. There is **no** therapy for this condition, a more urgent reason to explore every other possible diagnosis, Candida included.

b. Systemic Lupus Erythomatosis

This is another autoimmune disease demonstrating an array of symptoms: depression, fatigue, kidney trouble and skin rashes, the most classical one being the "butterfly" rash -- a rash in the form of a butterfly around the nose on both cheeks. It is frequently because of the presence of this rash alone that doctors start thinking about SLE. Many Candida patients show this rash on the cheeks and nose, because this area corresponds in Chinese medicine to stomach-spleen disorders. The therapy is cortisone. Not exactly what you would need if the diagnosis was Candida. We must mention briefly another skin rash often confused with Candida: seborrheic eczema. This form of eczema is located especially on the chest and head. However, by culturing the white flakes for yeast, Candida Albicans often is isolated. The rash regresses when the patient follows an anti-yeast diet instead of again using cortisone creams.

c. Interstitial cystitis

Another mysterious illness, its incidence is frequent enough to have created support groups all over the country. We already discussed the "cystitis" symptoms a Candida patient experiences. Urine cultures done turn out to be negative which makes the doctor think of a rare disease: interstitial cystitis. Not an exciting thought for the patient, since once again, no treatment is available. Whole books have been written on the subject, but nothing more than a description of the disease and some dietary measures are offered. The cause is unknown. I would like all the specialists treating these patients to look for Candida and CEBV. All the "Interstitial Cystitis" patients coming to me test positive for Candida and CEBV. Further, They respond 100% favorably to the anti-yeast diet and medication. My hypothesis is that because of the continous irritation of the bladder mucosae, after years of releasing dead Candida toxins via the bladder, the mucosa becomes irritated and will change subsequently to a rigid nonfunctional bladder wall. I have put the disease name in quotes, since again we are giving it a fancy name, describing a **symptom,** without looking for a cause.

7. THE UNIVERSAL REACTORS

Suffering from Systemic Candida might be a painful battle for most of the Candida patients, but they can count their blessings in comparison with the Universal Reactors. This group, about 10% of the present Candida patients, suffers from a sensitivity to everything in this world. In other words, they are allergic to the 20th Century. They not only react to cigarette smoke (a constant symptom of Candida sufferers), but to any fume, gasoline, perfumes, smell of foods, cats and dogs and everything around them (grasses and trees). The only clothing they can wear is cotton: polyester will burn and itch on their skin.

Unfortunately, it mainly hits young people (28-30 years old), and the bad news is that the number is rising and the age group is dropping. It will take only a few years before our teenagers will be hit in greater numbers. Imagine being a prisoner in your own home at that age. What can they do? More than ever they have to stick to everything in the therapy. One misstep and they pay for it with a week of discomfort. So if you, Candida sufferer, "can't take this boring diet" anymore, think twice! You would not like to trade places with these unfortunate people. The Universal Reactors always have the highest figures on their Candida tests, figures always double those of the average patient. Don't fall into the trap comparing yourself to other candida patients. If you gather a hundred victims, you would have a hundred different cases and gradations of the disease. Because all of us are subjected to different triggering factors -- hereditary, emotional, food and environmental ones. Anyone suffering from Candida, I strongly advise to consult my previous book on the subject, **"Candida, the Symptoms, the Causes, the Cure"**, available in health food stores and can be ordered at the following address:

Dr. Luc De Schepper,
2901 Wilshire Blvd, suite 435
Santa Monica, CA 90403

There is no doubt in my mind that at the present time millions of people suffer from Candida. The real tragedy is that 90% of them don't have the slightest idea what's going on and therefore are medically abused, misdiagnosed and suffer needlessly, losing many years of their productive lives. Therefore, I have included in this chapter the stories of several Candida-sufferers, extremely valuable, I think, since it will indicate that every Candida patient can show a different picture and even more importantly, that you can NEVER underestimate this vicious enemy.

8. CLINICAL CASES OF CANDIDA

1. Charles, doomed from birth on

Charles died at the age of 31 from a heart attack precipitated by cocaine use. Another victim of drug addiction? Yes, but as his history will show, it was very likely that he was an undiagnosed lifelong victim of Candida, which controlled his actions and directly or indirectly led him down this self-destructive path.

Charles had a shaky beginning. Six weeks after his birth, his mother was diagnosed as having cancer; she died before his second birthday. Her illness prevented her from caring for her children so the baby was passed back and forth between grandmothers. They meant well but did not give him proper nutrients and by age two, Charles was severely anemic.

He had several ear infections during childhood, each requiring antibiotics and by the age of eleven he had developed a serious craving for sugar, specifically for Coca Cola, which he would drink at the amounts of 6 cans per day. He also preferred eating out in restaurants to homecooked meals so that he could order his favorite food: steak or hamburgers with fries.

While in high school, Charles suffered from a severe case of acne for which tetracyclines were prescribed. He took tetracyclines for **14 years!** A bottle of tetracyclines pills and a current prescription were found in his room at his death.

There were other traumas during his adolescence as well.

His father suffered a severe heart attack and a few months later, he had a new stepmother as punishing as Cinderella's. Charles began experimenting with drugs to which he had been introduced by a "friend."

Paranoia, fear and depression dogged him in his late twenties and he began to seek professional counseling. He never stopped searching for answers. His shelves were lined with philosophy, psychology, and religious books. He loved music art and photography. The last six months of his life he put on considerable weight and remained aloof. The emotional support he had at the end of his life was from his sister. She was kind enough to tell me his story to help other people.

It is obvious that Charles was doomed from the start to suffer from Candida with all its ramifications. His mother's death from cancer caused him to miss the emotional nourishment of a normal childhood. Subsequently, the anemia, the antibiotics for ear infections and the tetracyclines for acne, lowered the strength of his weakened immune system. The immense cravings for sugar and fried foods were an early cry for help that never came. These cravings led to drugs to relieve him from his intense pain. It is tragic that Charles never had a chance to make something of his life. Everything went wrong from the beginning, there was no one to help him. We can shrug our shoulders and think that society is not to blame, but it is difficult not to feel compassion for this young man, whom we never understood. A beautiful life was wasted. Hopefully, this story will encourage parents to bring their children up in a healthy, emotional environment, with good food, few medications and lots of love.

2. Alex, 30 years old: a stress related case

When Alex called his off engagement in the spring, he did not realize that this would put him over the brink. He knew his girlfriend for over eigth years and had plan to marry her in the summer. Somehow he felt uncomfortable about it and decided not to go through with it. In fact, he did not feel too well since a couple of months. He was using cocaine and being in bussiness for himself, he was exposed to stressfull situations on a daily basis. At the same time, one of his bookkeepers was suffering from a full blown case of mono, and before they found out, he realized that on several cases he had drunk from her glass of water. Somehow, he could handle all this, until he decided to split with his fiancee. From then on, he was never the same. He felt extremely fatigued, had chills and fever and had trouble to get through the day. A battery of lab tests were taken, but all results were within normal limits. He was discouraged, because the fatigue increased, he became constipated, bloated and exhibited severe moodswings. His cravings for sugar drove him insane and his doctor kept prescribing him antibiotics for his sore throats. Finally, a doctor performed an EBV panel on him, and he tested positive for EBV in '86. A skin test for Candida turned also out to be positive. He finally was diagnosed correctly and could start his road to recovery.

It is interesting to note that Alex was doing OK till his painful decision he had to take in the spring of '85. However, it is clear from his history, that he was preparing himself for calamity. Daily stress in his work kept his immune system busy. The cocaine causes "heat-dampness" in the body, disrupting the energy in several organs but especially the spleen-pancreas (the immune organ) and the liver. In the past he suffered from prostatitis for several years for which tetracyclines were prescribed, destroying the normal bacterial flora. His encounter with the case of mono of his bookkeeper was another virus penetrating his defenses and threathening his immune system. Apparently the bigger emotional trauma of separation of his girlfriend was the ultimate depression of his immune system. It is a clear demonstration of the forceful negative impact of emotional trauma on the strength of the immune system.

3. Maria, 27 years old: a child of neglect and abuse

Maria's life started on the wrong foot: her mother showed such strange behavior patterns at birth, that Maria had to be adopted at age 6 months by her uncle's family. She grew up in the belief that her uncle and his wife were her natural parents. At age 5, her uncle's wife, which she thought to be her mother, died. Her uncle remarried when she was 7. This time Maria was less fortunate: the new "mother" turned out to be a monster, torturing her physically and mentally. To make matter worse, Maria was raped at age 16 by her step-brother. To escape the hell she was living in, she married at age 19 and became immediately pregnant. However, her unhappiness was accentuated by her immaturity which lead her to have several affairs. This lead to much anxiety and despair. She started to show all the classical symptoms of Candida, but was especially hit by severe allergic reactions to foods and most chemicals and soaps. Constant nervousness, anxiety and fear reoccurred to that extent that she is afraid to go anywhere alone.

It is obviously from the above that Maria lacked the emotional nourishment from age 6 on. The mental, physical and sexual abuse she had to endure lowered further the strength of her immune system to that extent that she has the tendency now to become a universal reactor. Her extreme allergic reactions are a sign of a hyperactive immune system, eventually leading to a full exhaustion of the immune system. It is sad to realize again, that this kind of abuse, so common in our society, lead to a destruction of life in its full meaning. It predisposes the patient to a weakened immune system, opening the box of Pandora to yeast, viruses and bacteria. May this example be a stimulus to any abused patient to seek help with a professional counselor.

4. Sarah, a medical calvary

Sarah, 50 years old, is a primary case of how one medical treatment can lead to another one. It all started with a Depo-provera treatment for endometriosis in '79. Alas, this treatment caused acne and her medical roller coaster started. Swiftly, Erythromycin (a classical antibiotic) was prescribed. To her amazement, shortly after that she developed a constant postnasal drip and constant sinus congestion. X rays revealed some air fluid levels, sign of possible infection. From the initial endometriosis treatment till the moment she consulted me in 1988, she managed to see numerous doctors, prescribing her the whole gamma of broad-spectrum antibiotics. Sarah, did not spare any financial burden, neither lacked the courage to seek relief from her progressive worsening condition. The famous Mayo clinic was consulted but at that moment (1985), all X rays for the sinuses were negative. A diagnosis of severe vasomotor rhinitis was made. There was even suggestion of tension, anxiety and a loss of self-confidence and self-esteem.

The next step was an allergist who found her to be allergic to multiple environmental agents. She was treated with repeated courses of antihistamines, desensitization and intermittent courses of antibiotics again. However she continued to have a mucoid green drainage and a subsequent culture grew some bacteria (Pseudomonas), but this was not considered a primary pathogen in her disease.

When she arrived in my office, after almost ten years of antibiotics, she was depressed, desperate, and sicker than ever. I did something what was never done before: I cultured the green mucus not only for bacteria, but also for Candida Albicans. And there it was: no bacteria, but Candida cells were found. It will take some time to correct ten years of unnecessary antibiotic intake, but she reacted favorably on a change in diet and the other proper measurements for yeast.

It is even obvious that the initial endometriosis was part of her threatening Candida syndrome. Endometriosis is one of the more constant present symptoms in Candida patients. It is a puzzle that nobody ever cultured for yeast: nobody ever considered the diagnosis. All these antibiotics aggravated her condition since they destroyed her normal flora, allowing the overgrowth of yeast cells. A ten years old mystery was resolved with one appropriate test.

5. Miranda, a victim of modern medicine

When I saw Miranda, 24 years old, in my office, I was astonished hearing her history. I thought I heard it all before but this case took the "cake." At age 23, she starting experiencing burning when she urinated. One month before these episodes she broke up with her boyfriend which turned out to be a major emotional trauma. An urologist was consulted who performed a cystoscopy, followed by some cauterisation of what was thought to be scarr tissue. The consequences were disastrous: she stopped urinating. After almost dying because of backing up of the toxines in the kidney, her urologist could recommend nothing else than putting a catheder in her urethra, three times a day. Of course, to protect her against infection, which is a sure thing once you have to cathederize yourself that much, she was put on a continuous intake of antibiotics.

When Miranda came in my office, she was putting this catheter in for already two months, with no hope of improvement. Her doctor could not predict how long she had to continue, neither could he give any explanation for this situation.

It is clear that Miranda went through the same insult to her immune system as many millions of people: the breakup with her boyfriend was sufficient to transform this outgoing sportive young person in a future victim of Candida. It is going to be an uphill battle from this point on: she cannot stop cathederizing herself which causes recurrent infections and intake of antibiotics, and therefore aggravation of Candida which was her problem in the first place. I hope to stimulate her kidney functions enough through acupuncture. Only when the kidney function will resume its normal activity, I have a chance to kill the yeast cells. Till then, it is two steps forwards and one backwards.

4

PARASITES, THE FORGOTTEN DIAGNOSIS!

Most Americans, -- including many physicians -- unfortunately tend to regard intestinal parasites as a problem related to poor, underdeveloped countries. When we think of these creatures with exotic names (Entamoeba Hystolitica, Giardia Lamblia), automatically our thoughts turn to such tropical and unhygienic areas. And indeed, that's where those conditions appear most frequently.

But let there be no mistake. As millions of Americans discover each year, we have parasites too. Many, in fact, are native to this country. You can get them without leaving your home, and contrary to what some might believe, they have no respect for socio-economic status. The parasites range in size from a microscopic single-celled protozoan to a worm that may exceed 30 feet in length.

Because the signs and symptoms of intestinal parasitic infections are often vague and confusing, and because many physicians in this country are not familiar with them, a victim can suffer for weeks, months, even years, undergoing many needless tests before the proper diagnosis is made.

Since the treatment of such illnesses is now much more effective than ever before, it pays to know something about these problems, especially when to suspect them and how to prevent them.

It is increasingly clear that parasites are able to take advantage of a weakened immune system to spread throughout the body, combining with other viruses and yeast cells. Therefore, they always will be in the differential diagnosis of any immunosuppressed disease, like CEBV and Candida.

1. COMMON PARASITES AND THEIR SPREADING MECHANISM

Roundworms

More than a million Americans are believed to harbor the giant roundworm, Ascaris Lumbricoides, which may reach 14 inches in length. It is relatively common in the southern United States, but can also be found in other areas.

It is contracted by ingesting the eggs of the worm, when eating meat, or from pet dogs or cats. More than 80% of the puppies born in this country are infected with roundworm. Children playing with these animals put their hands in their mouths and are thus prone to infection. Therefore, the best way to avoid contacting this parasite is to bring your puppy or kitten to the vet, for treatment beginning at the age of three weeks.

Tapeworms

Tapeworms are acquired by ingesting raw or inadequately cooked beef, pork or fish that is contaminated with tapeworm eggs. The beef tapeworm is common in the United States, the pork tapeworm is prevalent in Asia and Eastern Europe. Fish tapeworm is found in fresh-water fish in Scandinavia, Japan, Canada and Florida. The best prevention is to avoid raw and uncooked meat and fish.

Pinworms

Some 20 million Americans, mainly children between age two and four, are suffering from these small (half-inch-long) parasites. The parasite is spread by contact with infected clothing, bedding and toys, and by other infected children, who may carry the eggs under their fingernails and spread them to others directly.

Amoebiasis Giardiasis and Shigellosis

Giardiasis has reached epidemic proportions at this time. This protozoan infection is now known to be spreading throughout the United States. It has caused community-wide outbreaks in some places where the water supply is chlorinated but not filtered. Giardia also infects beavers and dogs, who may contaminate reservoirs with their feces. It is also a common cause of traveler's diarrhea.

Last summer the New York Times reported an outbreak of Giardia in a Montana town. It was attributed to water-borne parasites in the mountain stream that supplied the city's water. Because the parasites are extremely hardy, Giardiasis is difficult and expensive to remove from a contaminated water supply. One can add chlorine and let the water sit for a long time; or, alternatively a special filtering system must be used. Giardiasis is especially prevalent in mountain areas because the cysts survive best in cold water.

However, a major new transmission method of these Giardias has been identified recently in urban areas. It has been shown that this infection is significantly transmitted sexually, especially among the gay population, and it is this group that is presently at risk. Shigella, and the cysts of Entamoeba Hystolitica and Giardia Lamblia, can retain their infectivity for considerably periods of time outside the human host. Consequently, any type of sexual activity that includes anal-oral contact can potentially cause infection.

2. SYMPTOMS

Because of the generality of symptoms or because a lot of these conditions cause no symptoms at all, parasitic infections are greatly underdiagnosed. The doctor has to think about the possibility of parasite infection when, after treating conditions such as CEBV or Candida, some symptoms persist. If after an adequate treatment for CEBV and Candida, one has persistent gas, bloating and allergic reactions to foodstuffs which do not cause yeast growth, for instance, the possibility of parasitosis is great.

It is imperative for the doctor to know that parasites can be present in the absence of symptoms and a positive lab test. In fact, 50% of infected patients have no symptoms at all. Nonetheless, there are some symptoms -- unfortunately non-specific -- that can suggest the diagnosis of parasites:

- Intestinal, foul-smelling gas, worse in the afternoon and evening.

- A change in bowel habits. This is the most common symptom. There is a gradual, insidious development of intestinal symptoms over a period of weeks or months. There are soft or watery movements, or paradoxically constipation.

- Abdominal cramps and increased rumbling and gurgling in the abdomen, unrelated to hunger and food-intake.

- Weight loss in spite of ravenous appetite.

- Itching around the anus, particularly at night when the female pinworms crawl out of the rectum to lay their eggs under the skin.

- Food allergies, especially to foods that will not feed Candida cells (rice or corn, for example).

- A pneumonia-like illness, with cough, wheezing and fever, as well as a swelling of the liver. In this case, the cause is roundworms.

- Patients feel better after eating some food.

- For women, sore and swollen breasts not related to the menstrual cycle.

- Depression.

- Incomplete bowel movements.

- Chest pain, heartburn or heart pain.

As one can see, none of these symptoms is **the** isolated symptom of a parasitic infection. Most importantly, this has to be an exclusion diagnosis in **every** immune-suppressed patient. The combination of symptoms and the most reliable lab test available will provide the answer. If everything else fails, a short treatment with non-toxic anti-parasitic supplements or herbs will remove any doubt.

3. DIAGNOSIS

Until now, diagnosis of parasitic infection was made through repeated stool cultures (three days in a row) by a laboratory experienced in detecting parasites. However, the proper diagnosis was often missed because of falsely negative lab tests. Tapeworms are best diagnosed by finding eggs in the stool or around the anus. Pinworms are best detected by examining the anal area for tiny white worms at night about two hours after the sufferer goes to bed. Cellophane tape placed around the anal opening in the morning can pick up the eggs which are visible under a microscope.

4. ENTAMOEBA HYSTOLITICA

Entamoeba Hystolitica is the parasite that causes amebiasis. It is found in every country in the world, though its effects are more severe in warmer climates. It travels with enormous speed through the intestines. It is a microscopic vampire that can turn a robust adult into a feeble wreck. Amoebas have only a short life outside the host's body. In their dormant form, however, the amoebas become all-but-impermeable cysts that are amazingly resistant to chlorine and extreme temperatures. They can survive outside the body for a long time before being passed on to a new host, and they can probably be passed in stools for years by carriers who have a smoldering, asymptomatic form of the disease. In fact, the greatest danger is that some carriers never develop symptoms! Unfortunately, an amebiasis victim with no symptoms is just as contagious as one in excruciating pain.

Here are some sobering facts about amoebic dysentery or amebiasis. As many as half of the children in the world's least-developed countries die before the age of five. Of these children, most die from contact with food or water contaminated with excrement. One of the most debilitating facets of these diseases is the diarrhea caused by Entamoeba Hystolitica, which provides the "coup de grace" to small children already weakened by malnutrition. Through lack of sanitary facilities and clean water, more than two billion people are threatened by amebiasis throughout the developing world. These sobering data come from UNICEF.

You may be asking yourself, "What does it matter to me? I don't visit exotic countries." If you are convinced that amebiasis is an exotic import, you are dead wrong. Amebiasis is already a nightmare in this country. It is rampant in New York City, where half of the male homosexual population -- as many as 200,000 men -- may be afflicted with this disease.

Even if you are not gay or have not traveled to these exotic areas, you can still have been exposed, merely by eating out. Low-level kitchen jobs are among the easiest entrees into the job market for newly arrived immigrants. The job requires few qualifications, no knowledge of English, and there are no official obstacles. This is one of the major routes by which amoebas can invade your body. People in Third-World countries often become resistant to amebiasis but are at the same time chronic carriers. If a carrier finds work in a local restaurant and is less than scrupulous about hand-washing, he can spread the disease to customers. And be forewarned! This has nothing to do with the reputation of the restaurant. An infected busboy in restaurant "Chez Bigbucks" might be all it takes. So amebiasis is a major reason why "Employees Must Wash Hands" at your favorite restaurant.

Only recently has it been known that amebiasis is a "gay" venereal disease as well. The reason for its high incidence is simple. Gay sex is one of the few varieties of intercourse in which the rectum is regularly used for pleasure. Cysts (parasitic eggs) can be ingested at the same time love is made. And this is not the only way. Since parasitic cysts don't die for days, fecal matter can be left on the sheets, towel or mattress. This could transmit the amoebas to the next partner who occupies the bed. Fans of gay baths, please note that the Lysol spray used in the bedding and carpeting is an ineffective way of ridding a bed of cysts between occupants.

So a minuscule exposure to a parasitic disease will do the trick. People have been fighting this disease for centuries. But how can you fight a disease if you have difficulty in recognizing or diagnosing the condition?

Let's take, as an example 100 gay men, all of whom have amebiasis. Of these, 50 will have **no** symptoms, so they don't even think of going to the doctor. Of those who **have** symptoms, let's not forget how generalized these symptoms are: bloating, gas, loose stools, etc. Many victims will say: "I ate too much." Or "I drank too much coffee or alcohol." And remember, these symptoms come and go. So maybe with luck, 30 of the 50 patients with symptoms will go to a doctor.

Because the disease, at least at this point, is rarely diagnosed by doctors, only 20 of the 30 of the original 100 infected men will be sent for a stool test. Even if the best test for amoebiasis is about 90% accurate, only 18 of the original 100 will receive treatment.

It is my conviction that amebiasis is an overlooked major health problem. If we want to eradicate this immuno-suppressed condition, we will need all the weapons we have. Studies done by the Department of Health and the Gay Men's Health Project showed that 30% of the randomly selected individuals harbor protozoal organisms, primarily Entamoeba Hystolitica and G. Lamblia. Another study was done at the Cornell Medical Center, and again selection was limited to volunteering patients. The statistics were similar: almost 40% of the patients were infected with amoebas. We know that in healthy individuals, amebiasis is usually not a morbid disease. Immature amoebas migrate in the large intestines, living there as commensals, not causing any disease. However, with rampant epidemics of CEBV, Candida and other Herpes Simplex viruses, the immune system of those patients is suppressed enough without their having to suffer the ravages of symptomatic amebiasis.

What's the treatment? It is obvious from the above that prevention and a change of behavior is a must. It means cutting the risk involved in sexual activity. An interesting result of the parasitic attack is that it makes monogamy look very good indeed. Another step forward would be greater involvement by state health departments. An excellent step would be to require from all employees that handle or serve food to the public -- in schools, restaurants, cafeterias, grocery stores -- a stool examination as a condition of employment. If people are reluctant to have the stool test, a blood test is fairly accurate to at least detect the carriers of cysts. This only makes common sense: we have the opportunity here to limit a preventable contagious disease.

Of course, we have "magic bullets" for this condition. But as in other cases, the cure may be worse than the symptoms. At this point, Flagyl is the medically accepted remedy. It causes headaches, nausea, depression, disorientation and attacks of vertigo -- not precisely symptoms that will encourage patients to continue with their medication. And sometimes victims have to repeat several rounds of Flagyl before they can eradicate the amoebas.

5. GIARDIA LAMBLIA (Fig. # 8)

The fresh, fast-flowing waters of the mountainous areas of North America are no longer as inviting as they used to be. Skiing or backpacking vacations in the Rocky Mountains and parts of New England, where the water is derived mainly from surface sources, may be marred by a diarrheal illness; the agent most likely to be responsible is the protozoan intestinal parasite, Giardia Lamblia. However, unlike the acute bacterial diarrhea common to travelers in the tropics, the diarrhea resulting from G. Lamblia is not likely to spoil a patient's holidays. Symptoms usually do not begin for a week or more after ingestion of contaminated water or food, by which time the patients are usually back at home. Returning to work, however, may be another experience all to gether.

G. Lamblia is presently one of the most frequently identi-

Fig 8

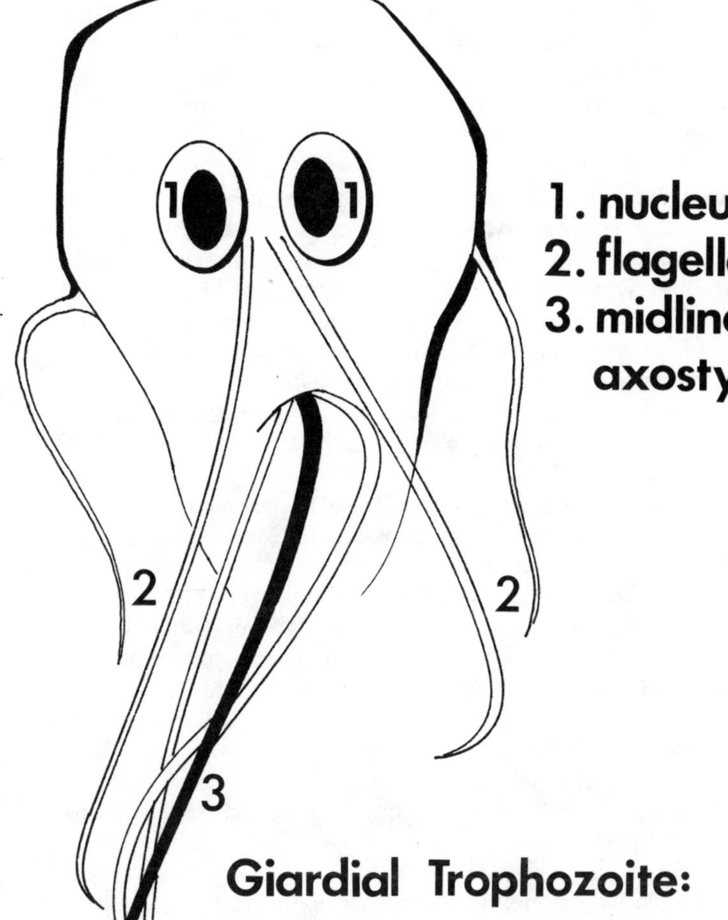

1. nucleus
2. flagella
3. midline axostyles

Giardial Trophozoite:

Frontal view, showing characteristic "badminton raquet" shape.

fiable causes of water-borne diarrhea in the United States. The main stumbling block in the management of giardiasis is the diagnosis. A number of cases are missed in the early stages because of a low index of suspicion by the physician; and even if detected, Giardia is frequently considered a harmless organism in the human gastrointestinal tract.

How is giardiasis spread? As already mentioned, it is probably the most common water-borne epidemic disease in the United States. It was not until 1965, during an outbreak in Aspen, Colorado, that water supplies were suspected as the source of giardiasis. Thus the danger of giardiasis exists in all areas where surface waters may be contaminated or where there is inadequate treatment of main water supplies. This can occur in remote, wilderness areas as well as in large urban centers (Leningrad in the USSR is a prominent example of this).

Giardiasis can also be spread by contaminated uncooked foods. Some people may be more susceptible to giardiasis than others. People living in areas where surface waters are contaminated usually do not contract the disease, probably because they have become immune. There is also some evidence that genetic factors might play a role. For example, it seems that people with blood type A are more likely to get giardiasis than people with other blood types. Gastrectomy (removal of part of or the whole stomach) and achlorhydria (absence of hydrochloric acid) in adults are predisposing factors to an increased susceptibility to developing symptomatic giardiasis, because the gastric acid barrier is lacking.

The symptoms are mainly those described on pages 151 and 152. Again it is important to remember that 20 to 50% of those who excrete Giardia cysts have no symptoms. The acute stage lasts from a few days to three weeks. Especially foul-smelling stools, absence of blood and mucus in the stools, and excessive foul flatulence in association with marked distention are features more characteristic of giardiasis.

How do we diagnose giardiasis?

It usually requires a high degree of suspicion, particularly if the patient has traveled to a domestic or foreign area with a high incidence of the disease. A routine question for the patient with diarrhea should be, "Where have you been?" If a history of travel is lacking, inquiries should be made about possible episodes of direct or indirect oral-anal contact.

The easiest, cheapest, and least disturbing diagnostic procedure for the patient is examination of the stool for cysts. At least three stools should be examined on alternate days before considering the results negative, as cyst excretion might be intermittent. However, failure to find cysts in the stools does not rule out the diagnosis of giardiasis. Since the giardia is mainly located in the **small** intestine, duodenal or jejunal (these are parts of the small intestine) intubation and microscopic examination of the mucosal biopsy are the most precise diagnostic methods.

Another promising test is the **string test**. A weighted nylon string is swallowed and passed into the small bowel. When withdrawn a few hours later, the fluid and mucus are examined microscopically. This method is a more comfortable alternative to small bowel intubation. The yield using this technique is about 82% -- comparable to the duodenal intubation. It is also less expensive than the three stool cultures.

If, at the end, Giardiasis is strongly suspected but tests are negative, an empiric therapeutic trial is worthwhile.

What is the therapy for giardiasis?

Although effective treatment does exist, no currently available medications is totally effective. Therefore, prevention is the ideal medicine. To begin with, don't drink the water from surface waters in problem areas (Mexico, New England, Rocky Mountains, USSR). However if you must drink the water, boil it for at least 10 minutes. Chlorination of water is not foolproof! If you are only going on a short trip, it might be worthwhile to take your own water. Adequate disposal of human and animal feces is essential to prevent the spread of infection. Do not allow domestic animals to defecate in natural waters. And, of course, avoidance of oral-anal contact will limit the spread of Giardiasis.

What are the available drugs?

- Atabrine (Quinacrine) is the one most used. Cure rates of about 80% can be expected; but adverse reactions such as nausea, vomiting, urticaria (an itchy rash) and psychosis, together with the relatively long treatment (at least seven days), make it considerably less desirable than newer drugs. The normal dose is 100 mg three times a day for seven days.

- Flagyl (Metronidazole), although not approved by the FDA for this indication, is the treatment of choice especially in developing countries. It is given as a single 2g dose on three successive days. Lack of appetite, nausea, abdominal pain and diarrhea are possible. A disadvantage is the overgrowth of yeast.

- Tinidazole is widely used in other parts of the world. It is highly effective as a single dose of 2g. It is available in suppository form for children. All these drugs should be avoided during pregnancy!

Although all these agents are rather effective, none of them is ideal. A safe, easily tolerated drug or supplement, which is effective as a single dose, is clearly needed.

It is clear from the above, that parasitic diseases are underdiagnosed and largely neglected. They are difficult to diagnose because of unreliable lab tests and, so far, are difficult and unpleasant to treat.

It is a fact that parasitosis should be considered in **every** immuno-suppressed patient. We have to realize that when our immune system is depressed because of other immuno-suppressed conditions, that parasites have a tendancy to flourish. Amoebas and Giardas are found here in the United States. New York has become a major center, and the problem will probably get a lot worse, as usual, before it gets the attention it deserves. If you suffer from Candida, CEBV, and Herpes Simplex viruses, make your doctor look for parasites. Your immune system will thank you for the rest of your life.

5

AIDS: THE SCOURGE OF THIS CENTURY

1. THE BEGINNING

AIDS will be the biggest test for compassion and empathy in this century. For some people, it is hard to imagine how they would react in the presence of AIDS victims. Others know for sure: they would have nothing to do with them. What is even worse, they would have nothing to do with the sufferers' families. Hard to imagine? Try to picture the following scenario, which could be common place in a couple of years. It might be you, living this nightmare. Here you are, a 49-year-old woman and your world has suddenly come to an end. There is only one thought in your mind: "How would people react if they knew that I am sharing a bed with a man who has tested positive for exposure to the AIDS virus?" You think you **know** the answer: they would avoid you like the plague, they would run, fleeing for their lives. Would there be a lonelier person in the world than you?

"You should have known better," some will say. They don't know that you just found out that your husband, to whom you were happily married for 20 years, had been leading a secret sexual life. "You could have left him," others will tell you. Of course you could; and when you thought of the risk you ran of catching the disease, you were angry and considered leaving him. But despite all the lies, you still love him. At moments you wish he would die, and then other times, you are scared he will be leaving you alone. You see the suffering in his eyes, the pain and terror, the insecurity. This is a man you have loved for many years, and this seems to be the ultimate test for that love. You wish he had a more acceptable disease, a condition that would prompt compassion, so that people would come up to you and comfort and hug you. You are 49, look 59 and feel 109. But the only thing to do is hang on. Your love ties you to this man. You take your chances that nobody will know -- that is, until death comes. Is this scenario intended to scare you? No. It is just something to think about when you have a few minutes. It is also a story that will become increasingly familiar in this society.

HIV positive means an uncertain future. How did this nightmare enter the United States? What happened, and why has the epidemic spread so far? Doctors traced the first cases back to 1979. However, in 1987 researchers jolted the medical community with evidence that the disease may have made its first appearence in the United States almost 15 years earlier. It was the story story of a young black man, 16 years old, who showed up at the St. Louis City Hospital with chronic genital swelling. Researchers found chlamidia, not uncommon in sexually active persons. But what was strange was that he did not respond to routine therapy. His muscles wasted away, and he died shortly therafter, leaving the medical community mystified. In the hope that medical advances might someday solve this mystery, his blood was frozen. Last year (1987) it tested positive for the AIDS virus, rocking the medical community to its foundations. Where was the entry point in this country? When and how early did it occur? Burning questions still remained unresolved.

What we can conclude from this is that the history of AIDS in the U.S. may have a much longer prologue than once was suspected. It probably was around for a long time but just was'nt recognized. It certainly predates the case of the Canadian flight attendant, Gaetan Dugas, who for a long time was considered "Patient Zero," since he was the key transmitter, responsible for the first recorded cluster of AIDS patients. Traveling extensively, Dugas was able to spread the disease to different corners of the country, making it difficult at first for scientists to link all these cases. However, his name kept popping up, and it was this that put researchers on the right track. The links bore out fears about the virus having a long latency period. For instance, some of the victims did not show symptoms until months after Dugas spent the weekend with them.

Since the AIDS virus was not epidemic in 1969 (when Robert R., the black teenager was diagnosed), it is possible that it mutated and became more virulent in the 1970s. If scientists are able to trace all the possible changes the virus has undergone, it might be that the puzzling case of Robert R. will be of enormous importance in finding a chink in the armor of the AIDS virus. The most significant questions we must ask ourselves are: "How has this virus learned to elude the 'radar' of the immune system?" and "What are its avenues of spreading and penetrating our defense system?"

2. EPIDEMIOLOGY: TRANSMISSION AND SPREADING MECHANISMS

A. SPREADING MECHANISMS

The invader is tiny, about one sixteen-thousandth the size of a pinhead. Its structure is very basic: a double-layered shell of proteins around a nucleus of RNA or Ribonucleic Acid. As in the case of any intruder, the immune system is alert and sends an array of cells to deal with this threat. But herein lies the danger. The AIDS virus seems to ignore most of our defenders cells, but zooms in on the receptor, found on the surface of the "General" of the immune system, the Helper T cell. It fits in there like the perfect key into a lock, and the door to our most sensitive and valuable system opens wide. The virus penetrates the cell membrane and strips the cell from its protective shell in the process. Within half an hour, the virus and its enzyme float in the cytoplasm, the fluid interior of the cell.

With the help of the enzyme, the naked AIDS virus converts its RNA into DNA (Double-stranded Deoxyribonucleic Acid), the master molecule of life. The DNA penetrates the cell nucleus, inserts itself into a chromosome, bringing into movement a new cellular machinery directed at producing more of these deadly viruses. Eventually the cell swells and dies, releasing a new flood of viruses to attack other cells, including more Helper T cells and macrophages. As you can see, the immune system gets stripped of its crucial defenders, the T cells, and therefore responds inadequately to infectious attacks. This is the moment when exotic sounding and opportunistic bacteria and viruses attack the body. Having reached this point, it is only a matter of time: the AIDS victim will succumb to his infections.

B. TRANSMISSION OF THE VIRUS

1. MAIN GROUPS

Acquired Immune Deficiency Syndrome is increasingly seen as a consuming global problem that may kill millions of people before the end of this century and profoundly influence human events well into the 21st century. From the nations that have already witnessed the suffering and deaths of thousands of AIDS patients to those where the disease remains rare, there is a growing -- although by no means uniform -- willingness to commit resources and to take measures against the disease.

What is the number of actual AIDS cases at this point? The World Health Organization (WHO) reported that the total may be as high as 150,000, the United States having the list of most reported cases, followed by France. But in places like Africa, WHO suspects an underdiagnosing of AIDS because of inaccurate reporting systems.

How many people are at risk? The world's population now is five billion, with about 130 million births and 50 million deaths each year. Only a small minority is at risk of contracting AIDS. Those at highest risk fall into four main groups:

Sexually transmitted group (mainly homosexuals)

Intravenous drug users

Blood-transfusion victims

Newborns

a. The sexually-transmitted group

The estimated 105 million people worldwide who develop

sexually transmitted diseases such as syphilis, gonorrhea or herpes are more likely to be exposed to other sexually transmitted diseases, including AIDS. In fact, the concomitant presence of herpes, syphilis, and also Hepatitis B will decrease the strength of the immune system enough to bring these victims into a group more likely to contract AIDS upon contact with the AIDS virus.

At this point, I think scientists forget to include one other major enemy reaching epidemic proportions: Candida Albicans. We have already discussed how this widespread problem is still ignored by the medical profession, giving the AIDS virus a good opportunity to roam through our weakened immune system. These facts might be clues as to why certain people seem to be less susceptible than others and why sex partners of some AIDS patients remain free of infection. Those high levels of exposure to the other viruses and yeast cells apparently cause a "chronically activated immune state," which may increase vulnerability to AIDS.

Looking at the above facts, it seems almost natural that the homosexual community was first to be identified in the spreading of this syndrome. The risk factors include multiple sex partners and the practice of receptive anal intercourse. Getting infected by sexually transmitted disease was an accepted risk for homosexuals. They went to their doctor for the Penicillin injection and off they went to the next sex partner, and most of the time, the next infection. If tested now, almost all AIDS patients suffer from Herpes Simplex 2, CMV, EBV and Candida, a reflexion of the damage done to their immune system. Viewing the behavior pattern of homosexuals in the 60's, it was clear that this group was heading towards a medical catastrophe: recurrent sexual-transmitted diseases resulted in a stress on their immune system, leaving them at high risk for a burnt-out defense system as we see appearing now.

Homosexuals form a very well-known group, but very little is known about the numbers and habits of bisexuals. But the available evidence suggests that these male "bi's" represent a new dimension in the deadly epidemic. Health authorities consider them among the most likely potential conduits for the spread of AIDS to heterosexuals, who may bed them or, as often happens, marry them, never suspecting that their partners are leading a dangerous double love-life.

Now just when the majority of America is becoming terrified by the AIDS epidemic, the backlash has begun. "AIDS is not the pandemic (widespread epidemic) its publicists would like us to believe, but rather a relatively small public-health problem, which is 'inflated' by gays demanding special protection." Before this mistaken idea infects the whole population, it is worth assessing what we know and don't know, about AIDS.

First, AIDS clearly can be transmitted by heterosexual contact. That is the main route in Africa. It isn't here in the United States where gays and intravenous-drug users make up the vast majority of AIDS victims. Only four percent of the 35.000 known cases are attributed to heterosexual contact, and this percentage has remained the same for nearly a decade.

Second, because it can take eight years or more from the time of infection to develop AIDS, looking at current victims only tells us **what was happening years ago**. To discover whether there is a "breakout" into the heterosexual majority, you have to look at who is now infected, not who has already developed the disease. The government is planning a national survey to determine the prevalence of the virus. But the study won't be finished for at least six to eight months. Another study, planned on the advice of Surgeon General C. Everett Koop, is HIV testing in a major college to determine the prevalence of AIDS among adolescents. But both studies will only tell us how far the AIDS epidemic has spread, not how **fast** it is spreading.

So far, we are not in for a rapid sweep into the heterosexual population, as in Africa. Africa, with its levels of promiscuity, poor public health picture and assorted sexual diseases, is still quite different. Unfortunately, an "African-style" AIDS explosion is not the only thing to worry about. The CDC (Center for Disease Control) never predicted a quick outbreak, only a slow expansion until, by 1992, nine percent of the 270,000 dead AIDS victims (hardly a small health problem) will be heterosexuals who are **not** drug users. Studies show that "only" 36 percent of

California women who were frequent sex partners of AIDS victims got the virus. But is that encouraging? I think that more than one out of three is rather high and that a heterosexual explosion of AIDS might occur in the future.

An interesting study to determine the odds of getting AIDS from a single act of heterosexual intercourse was published in The Journal of the American Medical Association (April '88). Dr. Norman Hearst and Dr. Stephen Hulley, epidemiologists at the medical school of the University of California at San Francisco, estimated that the chance of catching the AIDS virus from a single act of heterosexual intercourse with a low-risk partner is one in five billion if a condom is used. The risk rises to one in 500 if the partner is known to be infected and no condom is used. Then there is the middle group: one-time sex with someone who is not in a high-risk group but whose infection state is unknown. The risk of infection here is a one in five million without a condom.

b. Drug users

This is definitely the group that is most responsible for actually spreading AIDS into the heterosexual population, not only of adults, but unfortunately also to children. It is difficult to estimate the exact number of regular intravenous-drug users in the world, many of whom may have been exposed to the AIDS virus through contaminated needles and syringes. New York, especially with its vast population of drug users, has been hit the hardest. Heroin users are one of the original "4-H Club" together with Haitians, hemophiliacs and homosexuals who see antibiotics as magic bullets to allow them to endure one infection after another. Of course, drug users are people who neglect every other aspect of their health: no regular or normal food intake, no exercise and a total emotional instability, sufficient reason for the AIDS virus to penetrate their defenses.

c. Transfusion victims

The news cannot be worse. A letter from your health department has just informed you that "the blood donor involved in your transfusion was tested positive for HIV antibody...your blood was tested and evidence of HIV antibody was found." Chilling words that can become reality in the immediate future for some of the millions of people having received transfusions between 1978 and 1985. Not that the risk of contracting AIDS from blood transfusions is so high -- just one in 250,000, according to one estimate. In San Francisco, in its "Look-Back Program," the Irwin Memorial Blood Bank found only seven people who developed AIDS among 400 who received blood from donors who tested positive. Of course, this is small consolation for those innocent victims who received transfusions to save their lives and got a deadly plague instead.

How big is the problem so far? Six hundred eighty-three (683) transfusion-associated cases have been recorded through March of 1987. Nearly half of these incidents were in New York or California. Infants are apparently more susceptible to this mode of transmission than adults, representing 10 percent of these cases while receiving less than two percent of the transfusions. However, the CDC estimates that as many as 12,000 of the 34 million who received blood before it was screened may have been infected. The study on which the recommendation was based -- a study done at New York City's Sloan-Kettering Memorial Center -- caused panic among the population, who flooded telephone lines at blood centers. Health officials estimate that one in every 2,500 units of blood was contaminated.

d. Newborns

Transmission occurs perinatally, but whether this is transplacental or at birth, or both, is unknown. The risk that an infected woman will infect her baby is probably high, yet not clearly determined. According to the CDC, 563 cases of pediatric AIDS have been documented since doctors identified the syndrome in 1983; two thirds of the patients have died. While at this moment it is estimated that about 2,000 children in the nation are sick with HIV infection, the total expected number in 1991 of children showing symptoms of AIDS infection will be between 10,000 and 20,000.

Who will care for them? It is a fact that nearly all of them are or will be born into poor families where drug abuse is rampant. However, this is one class of HIV-infected people we can protect today: next year's infected newborns are not conceived yet.

Another major problem for kids with AIDS has been clearly demonstrated by some sad cases such as the Ray family where three hemophiliac sons tested positive for AIDS antibodies. Fellow students boycotted the classes, the school received bomb threats and finally, a suspicious fire gutted the Ray house. I cannot condemn strongly enough this cruelty, stupidity and these senseless acts of people harrassing innocent children. Ignorance is the devil's advocate here. What to do about kids with AIDS will soon be as commonplace a decision for school boards as which textbooks to buy. Because apart from the group infected by blood transfusions, there is now a second source of students with AIDS: those who have been infected since birth and, somehow, survived into their school years. And, God forbid, the next child with AIDS might be yours! A little compassion for these unfortunate children is the least we can give them, since the benefits of attending school outweigh the "apparent non existent" risk to others. But Americans are also capable of reacting with considerable warmth and courage when confronted with the AIDS-in-school dilemma. It is important for those child victims to be with their friends. Let love not be the hardest thing to get for these children.

2. SUB-GROUPS

Having discussed the four main groups of AIDS transmitters, we turn to more speculative issues surrounding the question of transmission itself: therefore I will discuss briefly three additional groups that have been claimed as transmitters of the virus:

Non-sexual Contact with AIDS-contaminated blood.

Artificial insemination and AIDS

The mosquito AIDS scare.

a. Non-sexual contact with AIDS-contaminated blood

It has become a predictable scene in the unfolding AIDS drama: whenever health officials announce a new finding about the spread of the disease, another wave of fear -- and sometimes panic -- spreads through the population. One of the big worries in this AIDS scare is that the population does not always trust the reported facts about the spreading of this condition. Hence, waves of fear -- and often panic -- spread through the population when yet another way of transmission is announced in newspapers or on TV. This is understandable when we see that for a long time public health officials claimed AIDS could not be transmitted from a single exposure to AIDS-contaminated blood. But hotlines were flooded with calls, health workers came in for testing, and doctors thought about changing careers when three female health-care workers had apparently become infected from contact with the blood of AIDS patients.

We can react to these cases in two different ways: either we panic and think this is a new mode of AIDS transmission, or we can use some common sense and look at the facts. Thousands of health workers have reported pricking themselves with needles used on AIDS victims, yet the incidence of AIDS among them is exceptionally low. What these three cases should teach us is the need for extreme caution. Whenever care givers come into contact with body fluids of AIDS patients, they should wear gloves, goggles and masks. The three cases described above were the first incidence of transmission of the virus reported in victims **without** a needle prick. But all these women had breaks in their skin that could have allowed the virus to enter. However, in all fairness, the risk to health workers is very low. Of course, as the AIDS epidemic continues to grow, even the small risk for care givers is likely to increase. In the near future, it might create another urgent problem. Some doctors and nurses, out of fear for their lives, could refuse to treat AIDS patients, as already has happened in a few instances. May compassion, common sense and taking protective measures against exposure to blood overcome fear, panic and cold-heartedness in the battle against AIDS.

b. Artificial insemination and AIDS

With more women opting for arteficial insemination, another (although infrequent) invasion path for the AIDS virus is possible. Yes, it is possible to contract AIDS from artificial insemination if the donor is infected with AIDS. Screening tests

AIDS, in addition to an investigative history of sexual partners are currently used by many centers working with arteficial insemination. Women contemplating arteficial insemination should ask about each center's policy to reduce likelihood of the spread of AIDS.

c. The mosquito AIDS scare

Just when people seemed about convinced that AIDS is not an easy disease to catch, some scientists have reported that there is evidence that the AIDS virus can be carried by the common mosquito. Even lice and flies have been implicated, but people worry mostly about the mosquito, which is by far the most common carrier of arboviruses. While scientists so far have never been able to confirm mechanical transmission by mosquitoes, some recent disturbing findings have raised new concerns. One of these findings is the transmission by mosquitoes of HTLV-1, a human retrovirus related to HIV (the AIDS-virus) and associated with T-cell leukemia. Another study, done at a private laboratory in Rockville, Md., showed that two days after feeding mosquitoes with AIDS-tainted blood, the virus was still found in the stomach of some of the insects.

Attention to possible transmission by mosquitoes was first drawn through the case of Belle Glade, a farming community in Florida. This community has the highest rate of AIDS per capita -- 375 per 100,000. What is important about these cases is that half of them occur among non-risk groups. So other factors must be involved: it has been suggested that the dampness and exposure to mosquitoes, and other, unknown organisms, could encourage infection with the AIDS virus. With everything that I have discussed about the immune system and its relationship to Dampness (which will decrease the strength in the Spleen-Pancreas), Candida Albicans has to be one of those organisms and, so far, largely neglected by the medical community.

The majority of AIDS observers reject the idea of mosquitos as a possible spreading mechanism of AIDS. They base their opinion largely on the pattern of AIDS infection in Africa. AIDS among children and elderly in that part of the world is mainly blamed on the use of dirty needles and contamination through transfusion. While I agree with that viewpoint, I want to mention an interesting finding from my practice. I am convinced that the presence of Candida is a major factor in weakening the immune system of patients. When we look at the age groups, it hits people between 25 and 40 the hardest, not so far, the very young and the elderly. The reasons have been explained before. Could that also be the answer as to why the mosquitos in Africa have an easier time attacking this particular age group and transferring AIDS in an already weakened immune system (i.e., weakened by the opportunistic Candida cells)? It would solve the mystery of Belle Glade, too, since Candida cells thrive in warm, humid climates.

The good news about the mosquito scare is that various labs show that the AIDS virus fails to reproduce and multiply inside the mosquito. However, I think that we forget to take into consideration the many factors involved in the weakening of the immune system, especially climatic factors, emotions and the concomitant presence of other viruses and yeast cells.

C. CO-FACTORS or "FAMILY MEMBERS" of the AIDS VIRUS

a. HTLV-1, AIDS's cancerous kin

While the desperate search continues for a way to bring the deadly AIDS virus under control, another virus of the same family has been lurking like a sinister shadow in the background. It is called HTLV-1, and it is the first virus ever shown to cause cancer in humans -- a rare and fatal form of leukemia or, less often, a neurological disorder resembling multiple sclerosis.

A study of drug users in New Orleans and New Jersey, run by the National Cancer Institute, found that almost half of them were carriers of the HTLV-1 virus. The target of this virus is the same as that of the AIDS virus: the T-lymphocytes, the director of the immune system. The origin of this virus remains a mystery. Dr. Robert Gallo, one of the co-discoverers of the virus, thinks it originates in Africa, while Japanese scientists traced it back to thousand of years ago when Japan was settled by central Asians.

There is good and bad news with this virus. The good news is it seems to be less virulent than the AIDS virus, and needs more than a single exposure. The bad news is that we don't know how long it can remain dormant before it causes leukemia. And it spreads by the same route as the AIDS virus: blood and body fluids and sexual contact, both heterosexual and homosexual. Just to be on the safe side, until more data are gathered, tests for HT-LV-1 are done by the American Red Cross for large-scale screening of this cancerous cousin of AIDS.

b. CEBV and Candida

Let the millions of people affected by these conditions not misunderstand my message. The above conditions do not necessarily lead to AIDS, if at all. What the reader has to keep in mind is that CEBV and Candida, are both immune-suppressed conditions, running on the same "freeway" as AIDS. CEBV, Candida, other Herpes Simplex viruses and more likely some other still unknown viruses are at the entrance to this "freeway," putting in motion a chain of events that leads to a continously suppressed immune system, with a total breakdown as a possible consequence -- AIDS. It is obvious that treatment of the above conditions is a must in the prevention of AIDS. Certainly people with CEBV or Candida will be more susceptible to AIDS upon contact with a carrier's blood or semen. The absence of such "co-factors" explains why some individuals, in spite of close contact with an AIDS victim, do not show antibodies against the virus: their immune system is not chronically weakened by other viruses or yeast cells.

In the case of CEBV, a new virus called HBLV -- for Human B-Cell Lymphotrophic Virus -- was isolated in Dr. Robert Gallo's lab. Although Gallo is not ready to say this virus is connected with any illness, I am convinced that it is a triggering factor in the CEBV outbreaks throughout the United States. HBLV is thought to be yet another member of the herpes family, but there is no evidence at this point that HBLV is sexually transmitted. To date, most of the AIDS patients have **not** been found positive for HBLV; it has only been isolated from those with B-cell lymphomas.

However, I suggest that scientists test their AIDS patients

for CEBV and Candida, and I bet they will find a high incidence of both conditions, higher than in the normal population. In fact, I have no doubt that almost 100% of the AIDS patients have at the same time CMV, EBV, Candida, Herpes Simplex I and II, Hepatitis B Virus and Entamoeba Histolytica. A study done by Loffler, et al., in 1986, showed the presence of Candidiasis in autopsies of AIDS patients in the mouth, esophagus and large intestine, as well as Candida abcesses in the liver. This information becomes frightening when we see that most young Candida patients, do have simultaneously EBV, CMV and possible parasites in their body. In my view, they are more susceptible to all the other infections, AIDS included, if they don't get proper care. Which condition comes first, we don't know. But there is the sense of a unique relationship between the group of immunosuppressed diseases (Herpes Simplex group, syphilis and Candida) and the AIDS outbreak.

D. THEORIES ON THE ORIGIN OF AIDS

As with any mysterious condition, many theories are being offered to explain the origin of AIDS. In fact, at this point almost anybody can come up with some theory or another. Since the virus remains a mystery, the question -- where and how did AIDS originate? -- leads to unresolved disputes and wide speculation among the most credible scientists in the world. In fact, even the basis of the theory -- that HIV virus is responsible for AIDS -- is doubted by some scientists. Peter Duesberg, an eminent virologist at the University of California at Berkeley, who has twenty years experience working with retroviruses, is one such skeptic. He reasons as follows: "The classic basis for establishing a microorganism as the cause of any disease is found in Koch's postulate. Two of the rules require that the micoorganism be found in **all** cases of the disease and that the disease be reproduced when inoculated with the agent. **Neither** is the case with HIV and AIDS! Once they said it was HIV alone that causes AIDS," Duesberg observes. "Now they say it is HIV plus co-factors. Until you can really define what 'something else' is, you are only speculating about both of them as the cause."

Ordinarily, a person is at risk until he forms antibodies against a virus. Yet with AIDS -- if we accept that HIV is the cause -- the disease progresses, paradoxically, once one has formed antibodies. The fact that the disease progresses in the face of intact immunity strongly suggests that HIV is not the culprit. It may well be that blood containing the HIV virus includes also whatever agent it is that actually causes the disease.

All this said, it is still worthwhile to examine the different theories in order to expand one's understanding of the epidemic. I emphasize that all of them are speculative and **only** theories, with the most basic questions unanswered.

a. The green-monkey-transference theory

This theory is probably the most popular one. A species known as the "green monkey" has come under special scrutiny. How this virus got transferred from the monkey to human beings is another question. A virus, STLV-3, known to cause a mild AIDS-like disease, was discovered in green monkeys. In order for human beings to come into contact with the virus, they either have to be bitten by the green monkey, or have monkey blood spilled into human sores and cuts. Neither of these transferring methods explains the explosion of AIDS seen in Africa. The number of people affected by AIDS surpasses by a wide margin the estimate based on the transference theory. Nevertheless, certain scientists hold to this theory, claiming that the virus underwent a mutation in these monkeys several years ago. However, the AIDS virus is more rapidly mutating than any animal virus yet studied.

b. The African -- swine -- fever theory

Another theory suggests a relationship to African Swine Fever (ASF), a deadly and rapidly transmitted disease spread among pigs -- and to humans -- by ticks. Swine-fever pigs exhibit symptoms similar to those of AIDS and ARC patients, specifically lesions common to victims of Kaposi's sarcoma. Researchers noticed that wherever there was a concentration of swine fever, there was a concentration of AIDS. That includes the Florida outbreak of ASF between 1979 and 1983, which may have been brought there by Haitian boat people and their livestock.

However, the mainstream medical community maintains

that ASF is not a disease that can harm man. The CDC tried to replicate previous conclusive studies, but found "no positive evidence." Nevertheless, many other scientists are critical of these conclusions and continue to investigate a possible connection.

c. Smallpox-vaccine theory

This theory was first published in the London Times in May, 1987. The reported investigation indicated that a popular smallpox vaccine was spreading the epidemic. The World Health Organization categorically denies this. The theory would, however, provide a possible explanation for the highest incidence in Central African states, since it corresponds with the most intense smallpox immunization program.

If all the previous theories leave you still baffled at the incidence of AIDS, you are not alone. There are even more theories, such as the Syphilis connection, the U.S. Biochemical Warfare research with the fabrication of new viruses, etc. I am sure more theories will be propagated as research goes on. Which one eventually will be the key to this mystery is as yet unknown.

3. SYMPTOMS

Many Candida and CEBV patients are convinced that they have at least ARC or AIDS before their diagnosis is made correctly. Some doctors contribute to this confusion, and in view of the similarity of the symptoms of the above conditions, it is almost understandable. However, according to their severeness, AIDS phenomena are classically divided into four groups:

1. **Symptomless** HIV-positive AIDS patients. There are no clinical signs, and there is no laboratory abnormality in the T4/T8 ratio.

2. **LAS patients,** or AIDS patients with Lymphadenopathy Syndrome. These patients show characteristic swelling of at least two or more lymphatic nodes apart from the groin area for longer than three months.

3. **ARC-Syndrome** or AIDS-Related-compound Syndrome. Patients show at least two of the following symptoms for more than three months: decrease in physical and mental powers, night sweats, increased transpiration, loss of weight (>10%), fever of unknown origin, diarrhea, fungi, Herpes SImplex, Herpes Zoster and impaired wound-healing. In this stage, we see frequently an increase in T8 or T-suppressor cells.

4. **The complete AIDS picture.** It includes opportunistic infections, persistant and recurrent, indicating defects of the immune system, as well as malignant tumors such as Kaposi's Sarcoma. There are several target organs involved.

. The skin reveals Herpes Simplex blisters in the area of oral, anal and genital mucosae; the Kaposi's Sarcoma produces nodes of red and black color in skin, mucosae, spleen, liver and brain.

. The gastrointestinal tract shows Candida infections being the cause of prolonged diarrhea (>1 month).

. The lungs are often infected by Pneumocystis Carinii (approximatly 60%). Other infections with Toxoplasma, Candida, Cryptococcus, CMV and EBV have been widely recognized.

. Central nervous system involvement: It is now clear that 30% to 60% of AIDS patients develop a syndrome of dementia characterized by memory loss, inability to concentrate and lethargy. It is a part of the AIDS epidemic that the public knows little about, and patients themselves prefer not to dwell on it. Scientists call it AIDS-related dementia. No one knows exactly how widespread this dementia is, but studies of autopsies show that 80% of AIDS patients have central-nervous-system pathology. And it is not just the case with adults. In a study at the State University of New York, 61 of 68 children with AIDS had nervous-system-related problems, such as spasticity, or the inability to learn to speak.

The mental decline in AIDS-related dementia can be gradual or precipitous, and it can strike early or late in the course of the disease. Ten percent develops dementia even as a first symptom.

This was slowly recognized by doctors, since AIDS dementia can masquerade as classical mental illness, simulating anxiety attacks, depression and also hallucinations. The virus' presence in the brain also vastly complicates efforts to develop an effective treatment for the disease. Any drug for AIDS would have to pass the blood-brain barrier that allows only vital components to get into the brain. AZT is the first and only drug so far that can handle this first hurdle. But whether AZT is effective once it gets into the brain is unclear.

4. DIAGNOSIS

Who is really at risk? Ordinary Americans are asking themselves whether it makes sense to be tested -- and what they should do if somehow the laboratory sends back an ominous message. However, many are reluctant about taking a test. A frequently heard argument is the following: "I thought about it, and for me, testing positive for the AIDS virus would be detrimental. I believe that the mind has the power to make you sick, and I don't need a reason to take the test until they find a cure." Unfortunately this opinion is widespread even among the high-risk groups. By avoiding the issue, one raises two questions with perhaps incompatible answers, one of ethics and one of emotional well-being:

- Do high-risk individuals have an ethical obligation to be tested, for the sake of past and future sexual partners?

- Does the lack of a cure make the test irrelevant as long as safe sex is practiced? Fear, of course, is the main reason why most people avoid the testing. I think that if treatment drugs were developed, one would see a lot more people coming in for testing. People ask themselves: "What is the advantage of the test, and can I deal with the results?"

Another hazard is the existent confidentiality law. Currently, it is illegal for doctors to inform anyone but the patient of test results. Under these laws, doctors cannot tell the wives when their husbands test positive; neither can they tell nurses that they are treating somebody with AIDS. It is clear that endangered third parties should have the right to protect themselves.

Questions about who should be tested, how testing can be kept confidential -- or if it should be -- and the medical, legal and ethical consequences of testing are piling up, with no ready answers in sight. It even has become a political issue. In the future, politicians hoping for election had better have some plausible answers ready. While this whole debate is going on, millions of already infected Americans are passing it on to many millions more. Of course, the best way to prevent this is to find those carriers, and warn them about changing their sex habits, and hope they will comply with this precaution. It is clear that testing has to start somewhere; but since it is impossible and too expensive to test everyone, who should be tested?

The government might consider mandatory testing for exposure to the AIDS virus for pregnant women, couples applying for marriage licenses, people seeking treatment for other sexually transmitted diseases, and all patients admitted to hospitals. The federal government now requires AIDS testing for active-duty military personnel, recruits and Foreign Service officers. All donated blood is also screened. Would this resolve all our problems? No. For one thing, even this massive screening would fail to identify recently infected patients, since it can take to up to a year before antibodies show up in the blood.

Moreover, if test results were made widely available, what would be the consequences? Perhaps discrimination in employment, housing, insurance, etc. Other questions suggest themselves. Are local gynecologists -- the physicians who would administer private AIDS tests to female patients -- prepared to counsel women who test positive? What course of action should expectant mothers take when there is a 60% chance that a mother infected with AIDS will pass it on to her unborn child? Abortion, sterilization? There is already a "hetero-panic," the fast growing fear among low-risk heterosexuals who swamp the test centers where the waiting period for tests exceeds nine weeks. Personally, I favor specific public education and vigorous measures discussed later, to halt the spread of the deadly epidemic.

What tests are available? The primary test is the ELISA test. About 5cc of blood is drawn, and an ELISA test detects any antibodies the body produces in response to the AIDS virus. Running the test takes about three hours. If the result of the ELISA is negative, testing stops, since there are almost no false negatives. Among the people likeliest to have AIDS, false negatives may occur if the test is given within six months after infection. Two positive ELISAs are the signal for a more precise test -- the Western Blot. In the Western Blot, viral proteins are blotted onto special paper. A specific pattern will appear on the paper if AIDS antibodies are present. After two positive ELISAs, a positive Western Blot is considered to be the final word. A negative Western Blot means that the person probably is safe -- to be sure, the tests should be repeated in three to six months.

However, in the euphoria of having a test available, the accuracy of these tests themselves has been largely ignored. There was a study done by the Federal Government's Office of Technology Assessment, which found that tests can be very inaccurate indeed. For groups at low risk, which will be the majority of people deliberately taking a test, 90% of the positive findings are so-called **"false positives"**, indicating infection where none exists. So nine out of ten hear this dreadful news -- positive for AIDS -- when, in fact, the virus is not at all present. Imagine the consequences! For high-risk people, on the other hand, we have the opposite: the test produces false **negatives** about 10% of the time, meaning that 1 in 10 of these people are told they are not infected when in fact they are. These margins of errors have devastating emotional and public-health consequences. They provide an argument against mass screening.

A new study on gay men in Finland also found that some who became infected with the AIDS virus did not form antibodies for **more than one year.** This is far longer than most experts had expected. The study was done at the University of Tampere in Finland by Dr. Kai Krohn. The new finding means that some people may have been declared free of the virus prematurely, before antibodies appeared in their blood.

The big drawback with the ELISA test is the lag-time problem: as mentioned before, it can take up to six months before an infected person has formed antibodies against the HIV. In other words, people who are actually infected, may be told that they are negative, allowing further spreading of the virus. There is some good news on the horizon: a new test, called **Polymerase Chain Reaction** (PCR), will overcome this major flaw. PCR testing test for the virus itself: it detects HIV within days or hours after infection. Two California labs have been licensed by the state to perform the PCR test:

Speciality Laboratories, Inc.,
2211 Michigan Avenue,
Santa Monica, Ca 90404,
phone: (213) 828-6543,

and the

Pathology Institute,
2920 Telegraph Avenue,
Berkerley, Ca 94705,
phone: (415) 540-1638.

Two groups are in my opinion favored to ask this test. Pregnant women who are worried that they might have been exposed to HIV since the fetus can become infected with the HIV before the ELISA test will detect a recent infection. The second group is people who tested negative with the ELISA, but their behavior--gay sex or intravenous drug use, puts them at high risk.

It is clear from the above that there is no strict rule available about testing yet. What will happen in the future is uncertain. Hopefully, fear and ignorance will not lead to two worlds in conflict: one that has the disease, and one that has not.

5. SOCIAL, LEGAL AND ECONOMIC CONSEQUENCES

A. SOCIAL CONSEQUENCES, or HOW ARE HETERO-SEXUALS COPING WITH AIDS?

Freedom, spontaneity, pleasure without guilt became the bylaws of the liberated '60s and '70s, as many men and women engaged in casual affairs and in relationships where standard moral rules were not applied. Today, with AIDS looming over the American sexual landscape, the situation is forcing partners to change their bedroom practices.

At first AIDS seemed an affliction exclusively of drug addicts and homosexuals. No longer. Although the numbers of heterosexuals with AIDS are still small, it is a growing threat. Right now heterosexual infection – among the sex partners of intravenous-drug users and bisexuals chiefly - accounts for approximately four percent of the AIDS cases in this country. Newly published studies indicate that the disease is bi-directional, that is, passed on by both men and women. As previously mentioned, a disturbing fact is that 90% of infected Americans do not know they are carriers of the AIDS virus. We cannot emphasize too strongly the necessity of changing life-styles immediately. To Americans in the late '80s and early '90s, that means a strain on any new relationship, since safe sex is the only sure way to avoid AIDS. Let's put it this way. It is hard enough to find attractive partners without having to quiz them on their history of bisexuality and drug use, demand blood test results and take appropriate security measures. It almost seems easier to give up sex.

Some think that this epidemic, this "black plague", is an Old Testament-style revenge for the liberated sex style we had in the '60s. And there is also reason for women to be alarmed. Women who are sexually active must face some hard choices. Often when they use the "pill" as a contraceptive, their partner does not like the idea of a condom since he is still not sold on the possibility of getting AIDS. I have a sound piece of advice to all women taking birth control pills (although I condemn their use because of the increasing incidence of yeast infections): do **not** tell your occasional partner that you use the pill, or you take a chance that your male lover will not use a condom. For him, the only thought is to avoid getting you pregnant, not how to avoid sexually-transmitted diseases.

Men seem to have other dilemmas. There is a strong reluctance to face facts. "I cannot possibly get it from this girl, she looks so innocent, she is so nice." "Somebody else will get it, not me." The ugliness of the disease is that we think that every stranger has it, not somebody we like or care for. Despite this concern, the quiet majority of heterosexuals in America apparently does not feel threatened. A recent NBC poll found that

AIDS has no effect on the way 90% of the population conduct their lives. People are in situations where they get aroused, and it is difficult at that time to think about what might hit them five years down the road. Adolescents, freshly discovering sex, are especially ignorant of the dark side of modern sex. The same is true for sexually active people at the peak of their capacities. But as more people get sick and die of AIDS, it starts hitting their friends. This makes them more cautious than merely reading about the disease in the media. People start thinking: "I knew this guy, I could be next!" So times are changing. Fatherhood and motherhood are chic, bars, one-night stands and multiple partners are out. The single girl, once the symbol of glamour, has fallen on sexually lean times, often deliberately. Attractive young women focus on career, sports and daily exercise rather than on sex. It is not uncommon in my practice to hear these women express deep concern about their sexual life, and many choose celibacy.

If you think that nothing has changed for the male population, you are dead wrong. In spite of the fact that female-male transmission of AIDS is much less common than male-female transmission (of 234 cases of AIDS in New York City, attributed to heterosexual contact, only five men were infected by women), many men are avoiding what they consider high-risk women. Terrifying as AIDS is, some experts feel that it actually might improve relations between the sexes. Often men lose interest in their conquest when the female gives in on the first night. Aside from sabotaging the possibility of a deeper relationship, casual sex is nothing but intercourse, and has nothing to do with intimacy and feelings connected to a particular human being.

B. LEGAL AND POLITICAL CONSEQUENCES

AIDS has been a subject politicians don't like to talk about, maybe even think about. Now there is no place to hide. Even for politicians, it is going to be the Number One issue in the very near future. The question "What are you going to do about AIDS?" is going to be levelled at them, and they had better have plausible answers ready. Will the panic be so widespread that "quarantine" will become the item on the political agenda, or will it be more financial support for research? Advocating AIDS testing for immigrants, federal prisoners and people applying for marriage licenses, politicians failed to get the support of many scientists and doctors. Controlling is not simple. In fact, nothing about AIDS is simple. Take the widespread testing for AIDS that our president advocates. Once the name of a person with the AIDS virus gets on a computer, he could find himself with no job, no housing, no insurance. A program like this will run potential AIDS victims underground.

President Reagan also told the teen-agers of America to forgo sex. We are talking here about the least-informed group and the group least willing to change their habits. So sex education should be urged. At this point sex education is offered in only three states, and only a small percentage of the students enroll in these courses. The rest learn their lessons on the street.

The president seems to be harking back to when family and church were supposed to be vehicles for sex education. But look at the number of divorces and the number of runaways and you can understand that for many of these kids, the word "family" is a phantom and church is yet another building in town with no personal meaning. Families pressed by economic lean times, or on the contrary, career-obsessed people, have no time or desire to teach their children about safe sex. The only way to reach this segment of the population is through education; and the best time is when they are young and IN school. The AIDS alarm bell has to be sounded in the classroom by teachers who are not afraid to be explicit. These children need to be taught before it is too late, because, apart from the homosexuals, the poor are at greatest risk. So politicians who would rather spout rhetoric about "getting the country moving again" are suddenly faced with the "Black Plague" of the 20th century -- a potential catastrophe with no cure and no political answers as yet. The U.S. Public Health Service should be spreading more "How-to-Avoid-AIDS" booklets; otherwise, the AIDS protesters, feeling doomed in front of the White House, will be the Ghost Battalion that will haunt the political landscape.

Rather than making the HIV test mandatory for people who get married, the government should make testing mandatory for homosexuals, drug-users and prostitutes, in other words, high-risk groups. In some states where HIV testing is a requirement for marriage, the expense was not worth the result: very few HIV carriers were detected this way. Closing of bath houses and passing a law that could give the doctor the freedom to warn the closest contacts of HIV carriers, would be other logical and life saving steps.

Aside from the difficult medical aspects of AIDS, this twentieth-century "Black Plague" brings with it a host of unresolved **legal** problems. Let's start with the first-line helper, the doctor. A physician may be exposed to litigation on different grounds.

Litigation grounds

- Breach of confidentiality. Disclosure of the results to third parties without written authorization for each disclosure is forbidden. Beginning January 1, 1988, however, a physician who has ordered the test may disclose the results to the person believed to be the spouse of the patient.

- Failure to order appropriate testing.

- Failure to diagnose.

- Failure to report the disease to appropriate health authorities.

- Refusal to treat patients in some localities.

Since mandatory testing is **prohibited under State law,** another problem arises. There is a growing number of inmates in California prisons who are infected with the AIDS virus -- as many as 3,400, according to some estimates. That will force the State at some point to designate a prison solely for AIDS victims. The inmate population has started to worry about this deadly disease. A film made by inmates called "AIDS: A Bad Way to Die," is shown now in various penal systems. But since sex and drug use are against prison rules, officially nothing has to be done. Prison officials pretending there is no problem are playing ostrich. Prisons are ruled by gangs, drugs are mostly readily available and anal sex is rampant. Ultimately, only fear will be able to make a dent in this stronghold of AIDS.

So where do we stand legally -- who should be tested and who should not? Ignorance cannot be used to rationalize responsibility. Everybody who tests positive must understand that he is a potential carrier of the AIDS virus and has a moral duty and responsibility to protect others from contamination. Certainly there are those who would prefer evading the issue to knowing the truth. However, a person who is at risk and refuses to have himself tested must behave as though he had been tested and found positive. To do otherwise is cowardice, compounding hypocrisy with wrongdoing. Moral responsibility is the burden of the sick as well as the healthy.

C. ECONOMICAL CONSEQUENCES

Surgeon General C. Everett Koop estimated that by 1991 it could cost Americans as much as $16 billion to cope with AIDS. It will be a heavy burden on insurance companies and on taxpayers. I am sure health-insurance carriers will adjust and try to avoid paying for services rendered to AIDS patients. The burden will be on the State, and it will be a heavy one.

Even the real estate industry is affected by AIDS. Last year alone, it cost the industry $1 billion in lost rents, lower property values and depressed economic activity. Fear of contracting AIDS could make it harder to sell homes or lease certain business properties in cities with large concentrations of AIDS cases. Furthermore, AIDS could deter some corporations from relocating to San Francisco and other hard-hit cities, adding to vacancies and lost rents. Fewer than 20 percent of major U.S. corporations questioned said they have policies to help employees with AIDS, although lower productivity and higher insurance rates linked to the disease could cost companies billions of dollars in the coming years. It is clear that companies, too, have a "Wait-and-see" attitude or simply hope for the best, which means it won't be **their** company going through this ordeal. Wake up, please! Not one company will be unaffected by AIDS!

It is clear that the AIDS epidemic will distort the economy

if the disease spreads as far as some observers fear. How the government will deal with this is unclear at the moment. Their hope is, probably, that a cure will be found before it becomes an economic catastrophe.

6. THERAPY

With no apparent cure for AIDS in sight, AIDS sufferers are easy prey for hundreds of quack remedies or doctors peddling half-truths and false hopes -- and potentially lethal treatments. I want to present here what is available at this point, while patients always should remember to adhere to as healthful a lifestyle as possible. Therefore, besides the following treatments, everybody, but especially immune-suppressed patients, should follow the rules outlined in Chapter 6 on treatment.

In the wake of this dreadful disease, even the FDA has eased up on some of its rules. There is a new rule now that will make experimental drugs available to patients with life-threatening illnesses. The FDA is looking for ways to improve the drug-approval process but still keep the safeguards. The authorities want to make sure drugs are safe and effective but at the same time they do not want to be so heartless that they lack compassion for those who are desperately ill and have no alternative therapy.

The major hope on the medical horizon lies in the possible development of a vaccine, the existence of some effective antiviral drugs and, above all, safe sex rules. As we mentioned above, it would be helpful to add to these treatments the necessary lifestyle changes outlined in Chapter six.

A. THE SEARCH FOR A VACCINE

Dr. Daniel Zagury, a French researcher at the Pierre and Marie Curie University, was the first researcher to test an AIDS vaccine on human volunteers in Zaire, Africa. Dr. Zagury disclosed that he himself was the first one to receive this vaccination. "I considered this to be the only ethical line of conduct," he told reporters. So far, Dr. Zagury has suffered no side-effects from the vaccination. In 30 days, laboratory studies showed that his blood serum was "highly positive" for antibodies against one major strain of the AIDS virus. However, none of the volunteers was deliberately exposed to AIDS to test the vaccine. This experimental vaccine was designed to stimulate a second kind of immune system defense, called cell-mediated response, in which special blood cells also fight invading microorganisms.

So far Dr. Zagury has suffered no ill effects from the series of four self-injections that began in November, 1986, and continued through 1987. He has developed what appears to be the strongest human immunity yet achieved against the virus. It clearly indicates that he achieved the expected immunity from the vaccine, which is hopeful if one compares this to previous experience with other vaccinations. The only thing that has **not** been shown is that it protects against the AIDS virus.

As American volunteers are being asked to sign up for the first experimental vaccine, scientists are wrestling with complex technical and ethical questions as to how to conduct such studies and protect the volunteers. Investigators will have to enlist thousands of suitable subjects, monitor them for years, and somehow prove that the vaccine is effective without exposing them to AIDS. To the consternation of scientists, they have had great difficulty in getting the necessary number of volunteers together, and some studies have had to be cancelled. But is this so surprising? Think about it. These vaccinated volunteers become HIV-positive, a stigma for anybody in the future. Are they going to be protected against discrimination in jobs, housing and medical treatment? Are they going to lose their health insurance, leaving them unprotected for any disease or injury? Who wants to take that risk?

In 1987 a small Connecticut firm, MicroGeneSys, Inc., became the first to win approval from the FDA to use their vaccine on human beings. Scientists have no evidence that the prototype, known as VaxSyn, prevents infection by the AIDS virus in humans. But animals that received inoculations reacted as the vaccine makers had hoped: they developed antibodies, that--theoretically, at least -- can render the virus harmless. But much remains to be done. Tests must be conducted to establish whether the vaccine has any harmful side-effects, and whether it really works? Even the most optimistic sources do not expect any vaccine ready for mass injection for another five years. Each stage of testing presents formidable hurdles.

First there is the mystery of AIDS antibodies. Most vaccines work by forming antibodies capable of defending our system against many disease-causing organisms. However, it is not known yet if an AIDS vaccination will follow the same pattern. Most AIDS sufferers do have antibodies to the virus, but do not get apparent protection, considering the progressive course of the disease. In other words, simply because a vaccine spurs the production of AIDS antibodies, that does not necessarily mean that it will fend off the virus.

Then there is the ability of any virus, and especially the AIDS virus, to undergo mutation, which means that an inoculation against one variety could be useless against another one.

Side-effects are another concern. Some experts fear that in the long run AIDS antibodies may disrupt the immune systems of individuals who get the vaccine. The good news about developing an AIDS vaccine is that widely different strains of the deadly virus share common "soft spots" that can be attacked by antibodies. It suggests that scientists may not have to make 100 vaccines against 100 strains. Quite possibly one vaccine can protect against many strains. It is encouraging, but we still have a long way to go. Most probably it will be years before we get a successful vaccine. Therefore, our immediate hope is medications that could prolong the lives of AIDS sufferers. A vaccine, of course, will not help those already suffering from the disease.

B. MEDICATIONS

While no cure has been found for AIDS, progress is being made in developing antiviral, immune-modulating agents to treat AIDS. The FDA has given top priority to all potential AIDS drugs.

RETROVIR, more commonly known as AZT, was the first approved drug for AIDS. The FDA's approval of this drug took less than four months, quite a record when normally years and millions of dollars are required to approve any drug. The drug was tested in a classic double-blind method, where 50% of the patients received the drug and the other 50% received a placebo. Since the results were extremely favorable, with fewer deaths in the AZT group than the placebo group, it was concluded that it would be unethical not to treat all patients. There was also less incidence of opportunistic infections and an initial increase in the T4 cells in the AZT group.

Unfortunately, as with most medications, there are side-effects. In particular, anemia occurred in about 40%, requiring multiple transfusions. This toxicity and the limited experience with the drug, serve to damp enthusiasm for the use of AZT. It is also important to remember that the long-term effects of AZT are unknown and that AZT therapy has not been shown to reduce the risk of transmission of HIV to others.

Several potential AIDS therapies are being clinically researched and are **not** approved yet by the FDA. Under the Freedom of Information Act, FDA employees are prohibited from publicly discussing the status of drugs under the agency's review. However, many of the sponsors of experimental drugs have made some information available. Isoprinosine, Thymopentin, Ribavirin and Interleukin-2 are just a few of those products.

Another problem researchers are attempting to deal with is the increasing danger of children contracting AIDS, when borne by mothers infected with the AIDS virus. Because the nervous systems of children are still developing, these young victims are even more vulnerable to AIDS-related neurological disorders. No therapeutic agents are currently available to prevent infection in newborns. Researchers at Harvard Medical School developed a surrogate model with pregnant mice and tested the efficacy of AZT. While AZT did not prevent infection, newborn mice lived longer and had a dramatic increase in survival. Encouraging also was the fact that the mice were born without any deformities. It is clear that a similar model will be used to test future anti viral drugs.

Attacking the AIDS virus directly with medications is just one tactic used by scientists. Another approach is to confuse this deadly virus with ingenious tactics. As already noted, the AIDS virus penetrates an immune cell (T4) by clinging to a protein receptor (called CD4). Once it attaches to this receptor, it has in effect opened a secret passageway past the "General" of our immune system, and the battle is lost. Scientists have come up with a cunning device: they have made copies of this CD4 receptor, and added them to test tubes containing both healthy cells and the HIV. The "imposter" receptors neutralize these AIDS viruses through a mechanism known as competitive inhibition. In laymen's terms, that means that if we put more CD4 receptors in our blood, the HIV will make no distinction between these "false" receptors and the real receptors, and therefore will bind to any receptor available, false or real. This way the virus is kept busy and neutralized. A drawback at this time is that we do not know if this form of therapy will help people already infected, with or without symptoms. Yet it is an interesting approach, currently researched by various companies. (See Fig # 9)

While extensive studies are being done for medications that kill the virus, other scientists focus on developing medications to combat the exotic and deadly infections that AIDS victims contract. Pneumocystis Carinii pneumonia, a lung disorder, is a classical complication of AIDS. It is caused by protozoa, a one-cell organism. In a fashion similar to that of the Candida cell, these protozoa are kept in check by our immune system, but go haywire when the system is suppressed, either by cancer chemotherapy or now in increasingly high numbers among AIDS sufferers. In a new approach by doctors at the National Institute of Health and George Washington University Medical Center, a combination of two drugs is used: an anticancer drug, trimetrexate, together with leucovorin, a protective agent against the toxic effects of the first drug. Many of the patients in the study actually recover from this pneumonia. Until studies are conducted on a larger scale, it is still too early to assesss the efficacy of this new therapeutic approach.

C. CONDOMS

A disease such as AIDS is a "marketing dream" for condom manufacturers. With the support of Surgeon General C. Everett Koop and even the Catholic Church, condoms are "in." However,

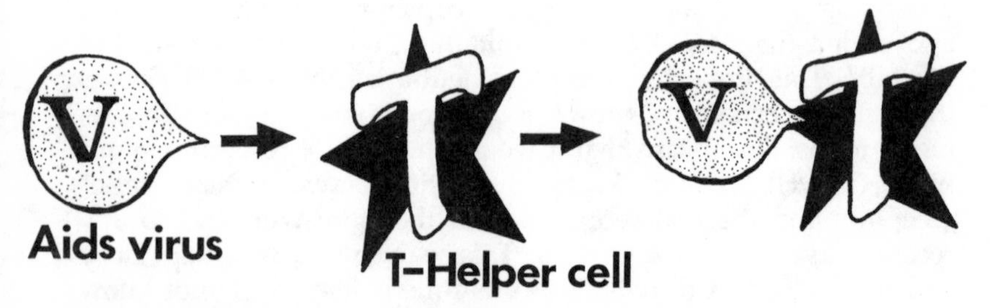

The Aids virus invades the T-Helper cell by clinging to a protein receptor.

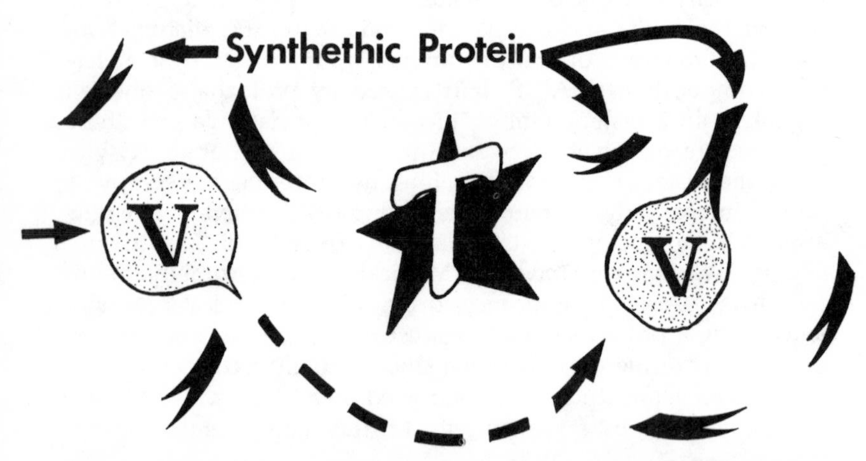

CD4 binds to the Aids virus and through competitive inhibition, arrests the invasion.

Fig 9

this form of safe sex is not as simple as it looks. Recent studies have indicated that natural membrane condoms are not able to protect against the HIV virus. For once, "close to nature" is **not** the best solution. Therefore, FDA allows only **latex** condoms to be labeled as suitable for the prevention of sexually transmitted diseases, including AIDS.

To maximize protection against these diseases, it is important that condoms be used properly. Following are some important and simple rules (it is amazing how little is known about them by the male public):

- Use a condom every time you have sexual intercourse.

- When you buy it, the condom is rolled up in a small package. Put the condom on over the tip of the penis as soon as it is hard, and before you and your partner get close.

- Leave about one inch of the condom loose at the end of your penis. That way, when you ejaculate, the semen will stay in the condom.

- Slowly unroll the condom onto the penis until the entire penis is After ejaculation, pull out immediately (hold on to the condom to make sure it comes out too!).

- Remove the condom, do not use again!

It is not a bad idea to use a spermicide with the condom, -- a contraceptive foam, jelly or cream. Since there can be leakage of the condom, and natural condoms made of lamb intestines contain microscopic pores large enough to allow invasion of the HIV, additional protective measures are not a luxury. Furthermore, condoms fail to prevent pregnancy about 10% of the time, a statistic that must make us wary of the transmission danger of AIDS.

D. ALTERNATIVE THERAPIES

Because of the lack of apparent success with any of the existing drugs, patients increasingly look for other ways to improve their health. Even doctors, until now mostly intolerant of any alternative approach, appear increasingly receptive to the idea. In this area common sense is the best guide. A genuine and humane approach would start with candor: "I don't want to tell you that it does not help, because I simply don't know!" I think it is the duty of any doctor to form a team with the patient, to inform him, support him and warn him against any "quack" therapies.

The therapeutic section at the end of this book contains many of these alternative, noninvasive (nondamaging) approaches. We already discussed the power of the mind and its link to the immune system. We should not be blind to the advantages of a healthful life-style. After all, only the strength of your immune system is capable of guaranteeing you full protection from these diseases.

6

THERAPY: HOW TO BOOST AND SUPPORT THE IMMUNE SYSTEM

Twenty years ago, how to strengthen the immune system was not even a question. Now the answer is the most sought-after secret in the world. It is evident from what we have already seen in this book that finding the answer is no easy task. There is no single-step approach available, such as we lazy human beings might prefer. Looking at the different causal factors as discussed in Chapter One, it is clear that any attempt to find a "magic bullet" strong enough to effectively boost our defense mechanism will fail. Another sad observation is that for most of us things probably will have to get a lot worse before they get better. Human beings tend to think that calamities happen only to others. Most prefer also not to read about the negative things happening around them, and even fewer are willing to get actively involved in causes -- for instance, the clean-up of the environment. Start talking about a healthful diet, and you lose 50% of your audience. "Eat that crazy food?," they ask, and "How can I give up chocolate, sweets and cigarettes?" Alas, there will be a point in their lives when they will run out of options: immune-suppressed diseases are on the rise at an alarming rate, debilitating millions of people in their prime. Will it take a complete breakdown of your own health before you decide that you, too, should make a choice between a healthful, fulfilling life or a short, struggling one, filled with the false pleasures of junk food, the willful blindness to environmental pollution, the overuse of medications as means to deal with daily tensions and minor diseases and a lack of soul-searching because it takes too much effort? It is your choice.

Only a whole-person approach can create the degree of immuno-competence that everyone of us will need to safeguard ourselves against disease. The strength of our immune system will mirror the health of our minds and bodies. I have mentioned in this chapter some powerful tools to be used by both healthy and sick individuals. I am confident that new studies will confirm what ancient medicine knew all along: you can increase the strength of your immune system in a surprisingly short time through some simple but powerful changes in your life-style.

1. EMOTIONAL SUPPORT FOR YOUR IMMUNE SYSTEM.

It is no coincidence that I start with the emotional part of our therapy. It is done intentionally, because almost all of us have the tendency to look for answers in all the wrong places: drugs, medications, alcohol, etc. Examining the deepest level of your well-being, your psyche, is painful. And frankly, you think you can't change anything about how you feel. How many times have I heard from my patients: "I cannot help it that I feel this way; I was born this way." Or "I have been this way all my life, and I can't change after 40 years."

There is a distinct difference here. If feelings overwhelm you because you have been familiar with them all your life, then it is time to get some help. What you are saying is that you don't know **how to help** what you feel, how to cope with those feelings. That is an entirely different matter. There are people who can help you control your feelings. In my 17 years of practice, I have always been amazed how patients who "can't help feeling the way they do" are able to drain my own energy in a matter of minutes. If I did not at once recognize their "dead-weight" attitude, in only minutes I would be dragged into that same ocean of discouragement. I have not been spared from emotional traumas myself, and I protested the same as anybody else: "Why me?" After all, I was responsible for this emotional upheaval. Just when I thought that I was ready to find peace in my heart, challenges, pressures, even calamities came up. And I said, just like a spoiled brat, "Leave me alone! I want peace and I want it **now**."

"Why are these things happening to me, **now**, when I really want to make some constructive changes?" It was a good friend of mine who filled me in. He said: "These **are** the challenges you have to overcome in order to find peace in your heart, because they have to do with your own unresolved issues. These issues are preventing you from finding your inner peace." He was right, and it was probably the best advice I ever got. Because realizing the truth of his statement made me calmer under heavy pressure, calmer than I was before when I had the false security of seeming to be in **no-pressure** circumstances. What I hope now, is that I can protect this new inner reality so that I can maintain the same sense of peace, no matter where I am, no matter what I am doing. Do not make the mistake of thinking that external changes can make you happier. "If I only could be in Hawaii." "If I only had $100,000 in the bank." "If only my boss would be nicer to me." Sure enough, a healthy environment is conducive to health and happiness, and a boss who likes you makes life easier; so might $100,000. But it is your mental attitude, that makes you happy or miserable in the long run.

Of course, it is ridiculous to suppose that a person can go to a two-day seminar and change belief systems that have been with them for 40 years. Such an approach only encourages stress-sufferers to fight symptoms rather than confront the cause of their stress. What such seminars **can** do is turn a person in a different direction, give them another path to follow. New directions are possible **and** necessary to change lifelong habits. It will take some time on this newly-discovered road before contentment, peace and harmony will be achieved. But is it not worth the effort?

Many studies have been conducted (and many more are yet to come) proving that thoughts and emotional states can affect the body's immune system. I see it daily in my practice. Once patients have gone through the original therapy for CEBV and Candida, for instance, relapses occur only when their immune system diminishes in strength. It does not happen after normal food intake nor after physical fatigue, but invariably after an emotional trauma. Divorce, separation, death or serious disease suffered by a close family member is almost invariably what causes reoccurring symptoms.

Not only do emotional traumas cause relapses, they frequently **are** the triggering factor for CEBV, Candida or other related conditions. Whenever I have a new patient, one of my first questions is, "When did you feel good the last time?" and immediately after, "And what happened just before that?" You would be amazed to see that almost 100% of these patients experienced an emotional trauma just before the outbreak of the condition. This does **not** mean that emotional trauma is the sole cause of the condition, but it is probably the straw that broke the camel's back. It is definitely the point of origin in most patients. It is almost as if viruses and yeast cells wait for the emotional stress factor to come and give the patient the coup de grace. It might be divorce, an ex-husband who remarries, an old boy friend who comes to town, etc. Even a happy event -- such as hearing about a friend who is finally expecting the baby she has been longing for, can and sometimes does depress the immune system.

We have at our disposal some tools to connect the mind with the immune system. **Guided Imagery** or **Visualization** is one such technique. It trains your mind to visualize health-promoting images; or you can go to the other extreme: you can visualize the invaders such as Candida cells or EB viruses roaming through your body. It certainly will help to put an image in your mind of growing yeast cells when you get those cravings for sweets, for instance. Visualizing how those yeast cells reach out for that food and start multiplying, killing all your healthy cells around them, will help to overcome cravings. Athletes create the perfect movement in their minds before executing it. Reviewing, for instance, a tennis stroke in your mind, before actually hitting the ball, will give you confidence and a feeling of focus. In the M.D. Anderson Hospital in Houston, Texas, young cancer patients play video games where they have T-cells pictured on their screen, zapping the bad guys, the cancer cells. It is believed that visualizing their enemies and protectors may positively influence the functioning of their immune system.

Combining fun and therapy to enhance our defense mechanisms can take other forms. Many people, for example, have experienced the beneficial effects that artistic creativity has on patients' recovery from cancer. By immersing themselves in something they love to do, they ease their pain and bring beauty back into their lives. To balance the loss of quality in life and grieving that comes with immuno-suppressed diseases, writing a book, painting, sculpturing or playing a musical instrument are as important as any form of therapy. Actually, for many individuals, these dark years, when they were confined to their homes, proved to be the turning point of their lives. There was no choice: they had to slow down considerably because they had no energy left; they had barely enough energy to survive. The generative force that comes with creativity proves to people that they can not only fight for their survival, but also that they can have a full life after receiving treatment. Concentrating on art, brings those patients back to an inner calm and peace, so much more conducive to healing than the rage and indignation to which so many victims succumb.

It is important for all of us to realize that **we** are in charge of our feelings; our minds do what we program them to do. We can either program ourselves with self-imposed limitations that keep us from reaching our full potential, or we can fill our mind with good feelings about ourselves. You have to love yourself before you can love anybody else. Since your mind seems to be at work all the time anyway, why not switch it to this positive mental program? It can be meditation, self-hypnosis or imagery; it all boils down to the same result: our minds become focused and take full control of our bodies. Don't fall into the trap of negative self-suggestion, where you tell yourself that you are too stupid, too clumsy or too limited to do well in a certain field. Take tennis, for instance. I am an ardent tennis player and know at first hand what a powerful mental game it is. Tell yourself that you are no good at it, get angry at yourself for each missed ball, and you will be surprised to find out that the game becomes torture instead of pleasure. Telling yourself repeatedly about your shortcomings destroys any talent that you may have. I see it often with my tennis opponents -- how they get into a low-self-esteem roll, just like a snowball rolling down a hill, incapable of stopping until it explodes against a rock or tree, which in tennis translates into smashing the racket onto the court. As you can see, telling yourself that you are inadequate and worthless will work -- but against you. So please imagine yourself more as a winner, not only on the tennis court but in any life situation. Just start acting like a winner and before you know it, you will **be** one.

When you discover how great it feels to be a winner, to be in control of your body, you might also find out how very refreshing and comforting it feels to use the power of your mind. So set your goals, try to determine what you want to accomplish, and go for it. If you don't have a mission, your mind will be in chaos, unable to guide your body in reaching those goals. Don't act like some of my patients who are almost afraid to find out that they have something wrong with them, because they do not want to change anything in their life-style. As one of them said, "Okay, I will follow this diet, but how many frozen yoghurts am I allowed?" My answer was simple: "As many times as you want to feel sick." These patients are simply not sick **enough!** They have to hit rock bottom before they realize that an immuno-suppressed condition is no laughing matter.

Biofeedback is another mental tool that can speed recovery. Biofeedback is routinely used for conditions such as migraines and stress, but it also has been applied in psychotherapy. It has been successfully used in cases of "multiple personalities", a condition where there are up to twenty different personalities inhabiting one body. This condition dates back to childhood traumas, severe enough for the child to escape into these different personalities to deal with the different traumas. The common denominator for this syndrome is child abuse.

Positive imagery and biofeedback are two tools that every victim of CEBV, Candida, cancer, etc. can use. Support from family and friends is another positive mental aid. Alas, while cancer patients often find the support they need, Candida, CEBV or AIDS patients are more often rejected because of ignorance or simply fear. Feeling isolated from their loved ones, not being taken seriously by their doctors and closest family members will bring these victims to a state of anger and depression. It is not only doubt that disconnects family members from the victim. It is also not knowing what to do, feeling at a loss as to why their loved ones are behaving as they are. Consider this: the doctor thinks there is nothing wrong with the patient. Lab tests "prove" it. (Of course, it is very difficult to prove an illness when your doctor either does not think of a certain condition or does not believe that a certain condition exists. So the **right** lab tests are **not** requested). I know at first hand how difficult it might be to live with an immuno-suppressed patient (See my personal account, "Open letter to the family members of an Environment-Sensitive Patient"). However, when we choose to be with somebody, we choose to be with that person for better **and** for worse. Finding this unconditional love is not easy, but it is worth it. The person who will find the most richness in this, is the one who can give unconditional love. How would you like to be on the other side, feeling left out?

I believe that, more than the lack of medication or a bad diet, negative feelings will depress the immune system and are responsible for the many relapses we see in these patients. It is incredible how many relationships and marriages have been broken up because of a lack of understanding and sympathy with the victims of these conditions. It is essential to realize that if the body is going to heal, then **emotional and psychological support are crucial.**

2. IS THERE A DIETARY SOLUTION FOR THE IMMUNE SYSTEM?

It is frightening to see how very few doctors are acquainted with nutrition. It is simply not part of medical training. I believe it is one of our biggest shortcomings in medical schools. Claiming that nutrition will not play a role in the maintenance of health, and therefore also the immune system, is like saying that it does not matter what fuel we put in our cars. I cannot understand why, with all the breakthroughs we have made in medical science and the intellectual power we are able to develop, our profession seems to neglect this particular aspect of health. While we sometimes have little control over environmental "food," at least we have control, if we wish, over the intake of our food. Alas! At least 80% of Americans have an inadequate diet, mainly out of ignorance or laziness. And there seems to be no improvement in sight. Radiation of food is proposed, and there seems no end to the use of preservatives, coloring substances or antibiotics in the preparation of foods. Only awareness and a boycott of these foods will bring the sorely needed changes. I think that diseases such as CEBV, Candida and other related immune-suppressed diseases will force these changes.

Are there foods that would help maintain the strength of the immune system? Or is this just "quackery" as some claim? The promotion of long life and good health through diet is no longer supported solely by folk wisdom and pseudo-science. Since 1980, the National Cancer Institute (NCI) has advocated research into whether diet can protect people from cancer. And if we mention cancer, the ultimate destruction of our immune system, we cannot be impervious to the results of these studies in terms of the beneficial effect they may have on other immune-suppressed diseases. Even though many of the NCI studies won't be finished for several years, the picture is already clear enough to conclude that ALL of us can benefit from dietary changes.

I have depicted the many unnecessary and deleterious changes we made in our foods in Chapter One. I will be blunt: the best start you can make for your dietary changes is by shopping **solely** in health food stores. Have you tried to find foods that contain no preservatives, sugar, coloring substances, hormones or antibiotics in your local supermarket? This is nearly impossible. Sometimes there is a small separate section for "Health Foods." Isn't it ironic? What then are we going to call all the other products? "Unhealthy" foods? We should call them just that -- because most of them actually are. Many patients have no choice anymore. They **have** to buy foods in the health food stores because they will have reactions to anything they buy in regular markets. These might constitute a small percentage of consumers still, but they are growing in number. Let food not be the factor that makes you sick; there are more than enough other immune-suppressing factors threatening you.

A good example of an immune-stimulating diet is the "Candida diet" outlined in Chapter Three. However, for a healthy individual to maintain health, certain restrictions for Candida patients are not applicable. The diet can be more liberal, although the principles are the same. Combining the knowledge of toxic factors in food, as outlined in Chapter One, with a diet such as the Candida one, will put you instantly on the right track. What I will add here are some important food facts and some more information about food composition. Inevitably we will need to discuss the supplements required to support our immune system. "Superfoods" are often considered "super" because they contain essential elements such as beta carotene, selenium, Vitamin C, etc., antioxidants, and main fuel for our defense system.

a. The neglected nutrient of modern times: fiber

Fiber is a broad term covering a complex mixture of many substances. Initially it was defined as roughage of plants after the digestive process. Recently fibers also include some substances such as pectins, gums and mucilages found in many fruits. Fiber is not absorbed by the body and thus is not defined as one of the essential nutrients, requiring minimum daily requirements. And that's where our problem starts.

Americans have diets that are abnormally low in fiber. We should increase our intake to 30 grams of fiber a day, depending on our size (larger individuals should consume more). One of the facts attracting more attention to increased use of fiber was President's Reagan colon cancer. The media highlighted causes and brought the discussion of early detection and prevention into broad daylight. Because of the patient involved, many people changed their habits (and I hope not temporarily). Fiber not only plays a role in the prevention of colon cancer, but equally important in the prevention of arteriosclerosis and increased cholesterol levels, two factors linked to cardiovascular disease. This affects not only adults. In the Vietnam war, autopsies were performed on young victims (18-year-olds), and to the amazement of pathologists, sometimes extensive arteriosclerosis was found in their vessels. It does not surprise me. American kids get an average of 40% of their calories from fat, and they have the artery scars to show for it. Look at the major part of kids' food intake: potato chips, cookies, white bread, French fries, red meat, colas, candy, ice cream, etc. No wonder early coronary disease is documented more and more in young accident, homicide or suicide victims; and it is in direct proportion to their cholesterol levels. While adults' cholesterol level should be below 230 milligrams, a cholesterol count of even 150 mgs is considered too high for children. So please, parents, since the burden for preventing future heart attacks is increasingly falling upon you, add fruits, vegetables and cereals (without sugar) to the diets of your children.

b. Beta Carotene

Beta carotene has always been considered a frontrunner in the defense of our immune system. What is this precious nutrient? It is the precursor of Vitamin A, a "Provitamin." While Vitamin A consumption has restrictions (it is one of the only vitamins that can be toxic in overuse), beta carotene is safe. There is a security system: beta carotene is converted to Vitamin A as it is needed by the body. Even taken in high doses, it is harmless. Mostly one notes the appearance of yellow palms and soles.

For a long time we have known the benefits of Vitamin A provided by beta carotene: improved night vision, growth of teeth, nails and hair. But beta carotene is one of the most powerful antioxidants; in other words, it protects our cells against harmful elements in our environment. Apparently beta carotene has even attracted the attention of the National Cancer Institute. A study sponsored at Harvard Medical School suggested enough evidence that foods rich in beta carotene reduce the risk of cancer.

Does this mean that all of us should run to the health food store and start supplementing our diets with this miracle nutrient? It depends on your diet. Surveys have shown that the majority of the American people do not receive the recommended levels of Vitamin A. Judge for yourself. Do you eat enough foods such as carrots, spinach, sweet potatoes, parsley, kale and collards? If not, you belong to the majority. Therefore, supplementing with extra beta carotene, especially in light of its non-toxicity, is advised. Take 25.000 Units of beta carotene, twice a day. Another supplement, **Spirulina,** has attracted attention in this context. It is an extract of blue-green algae of which beta carotene is a major component. Besides beta carotene, it contains many other carotenoids. The functions of the latter are still unknown, but they probably work in a synergistic way with beta carotene and Vitamin E, another powerful antioxidant. Many studies are still under way, but so far we may presume that beta carotene will be a major soldier in our immune system.

c. Vitamin E foods

More and more people are victimized by the environment.

What is more frightening, the victims seem to be getting younger and younger. Twenty-year-old patients are incapable of going many places, because they react to gasoline fumes, perfumes, building materials, gas, and polyester clothing. They get sick in their own cars, making them totaly housebound. Not is this rarity any longer. It is becoming more and more commonplace. Moreover, the problem is going to get a lot worse before it gets better. Since we cannot change our environment immediately, we need to protect ourselves with Vitamin E, a potent antioxidant, which has a proven ability to protect cell membranes against chemical damage.

Women especially seem to be victims of a lack of this precious vitamin. Since estrogen destroys Vitamin E, the popular overuse of "the pill" leaves them with even less of this nutrient in their bodies. Since smoking has increased in women since the 60's (smoking decreases the Vitamin E level) and many women are overweight, extra E is advisable.

Food is not really a good supplier. You can find Vitamin E in eggs, spinach and cold-pressed cottonseed oil. With the tendency to omit eggs from the diet because of the cholesterol scare, it does not look like the average American will get much of the 400 I.U. Vitamin E needed per day. So supply yourself with 400 I.U. of Vitamin E daily. In case of fibrocystic disease of the breast, a dosis of 800 I.U. daily has been shown to remedy the condition in 80% of the cases. Chances of conquering fibrocystic disease increase when Evening Primrose Oil is added (4 capsules daily).

d. Vitamin C foods

Linus Pauling, Ph.D., winner of 2 Nobel prizes, is in my view one of the last geniuses of this century. Amazingly enough, in spite of his research, most of the medical establishment never use Vitamin C in their practices. When you suggest giving large quantities intravenously, they try to convince you that you take a risk in developing kidney stones.

However, by focussing on that particular effect which by no means is proven, you miss out a lot. There is nothing better than high doses of Vitamin C for common colds. In the case of flu, our first reaction should be high intake of Vitamin C, 1 tsp. buffered

C powder, every other hour. If loose stools result, decrease the intake. Vitamin C is certainly one of the biggest aids in the treatment of CEBV and Candida. A Vitamin C drip will boost these patients' energy and spirit until the rest of the treatment has taken effect. It is not uncommon at all for patients to take up to 25 **grams** of Vitamin C, a far cry from the recommended RDA dosage of 500 **milligrams**. In any case, a minimum of 4-6000 mgs is advised for anybody who wants to boost their immune system. Nature provides a lot of Vitamin C: citrus fruits, berries, potatoes, tomatoes, cauliflower, corn and sagopalm. One thing to keep in mind when administering high doses of Vitamin C: some people are allergic to corn and I have not found yet an intravenously available product derived from hiprose or sagopalm or potato. Most people have no problem with the corn-derived Vitamin C, but a minority will have strong allergic reactions, enhanced by the intravenous injection.

e. Zinc foods

It is known that the thymus, behind the breastbone, grows from birth till puberty. From then on, it will only shrink in size. Since the thymus is the production place of the T-cells, this will limit their number. By supplementing one's diet with 50 mgs zinc, especially the orothate form, we will effectively bolster the thymus. Zinc is commonly deficient in the American diet, especially among the elderly, who need it the most. Since intake of extra Zinc can cause gastric discomfort, it is best to take it after meals. Natural sources of zinc are round steak, pork, pumpkin seeds, eggs and mustard.

f. Coenzyme Q10

As with many other supplements first brought to the attention of the public, Coenzyme Q10 has been hailed as a miracle nutrient. It is an important "co-worker" of the enzymes that guide the complicated biochemical reactions in our body. Every functioning cell in the body will be influenced by the presence of Coenzyme Q10. A lack of it will make these reactions sluggish and the cells will function at a decreased rate, initiating an array of diseases. It has been found that immuno-suppressed patients have low levels of Coenzyme Q10. Moreover it takes its place with the antioxidants – Vitamin E, Vitamin C and Selenium – in protecting our cells against damaging free radicals.

It would seem to be wise to add to your potential of "soldiers" about 60 to 100 mgs Coenzyme Q10.

g. Germanium

The word "miracle" seems to pop up constantly whenever a new supplement is introduced. Unfortunately, it also comes with "black market" pricing and all kinds of inferior-quality products. Patients simply no longer know what to look for; fancy names and dosages on the labels add to the confusion, and the potential for fraud is increased.

I certainly think, this was not Dr. Kazuhiko Asai's goal, when he catapulted Germanium into the limelight. This brilliant man, who has founded the Germanium institute in Japan, has dedicated his life to bringing the world the medical benefits of germanium.

The existence of the Element Germanium was already foreseen by Dmitri Mendeleev, the Russian chemist who put together the periodic table of elements. Later on, Germanium received little attention until Dr. Kazuhiko Asai Ph.D., who established the Coal Center Foundation in Japan, focused his attention on the presence of Germanium found in coal. He developed a process whereby he removed the germanium from coal, and started to use it first on himself, later on other people to help them recovering from different ailments. The rest is history. The apparent results drew enough attention to the American consumer that it became a household word in many families.

If you are looking for the "real" thing, you had better check the labels for "organic" Germanium or Sesquioxyde Germanium. It is available in different forms: powder, capsules and ampoules. Doses seem to vary according to the condition. For our Candida and CEBV patients, 250-500mgs daily are advised. If you take the powder, which will be the most economical, it is better to divide the doses over different times of the day. It is also beneficial to hold the powder under the tongue, since absorption in the blood will be enhanced.

Germanium simply provides us with more oxygen, therefore giving the body the opportunity to fight disease by its own powers. As with the other immuno suppressed diseases, an alkaline diet (more fish, grains and vegetables, and less meat) is basic. A well-balanced diet is **the** beginning point of any health plan.

h. Polyzym 22

This is an original product from Germany, produced by MUCOS Pharma GmbH, bought in Germany under the name WOBE-MUGOS and Polyzym O22 here in the USA (GRL). It is composed of Trypsin of pancreas 40 mg, Chymotrypsin of pancreas 40 mg, Papainases 100 mg and Thymus 40 mg. As one can see, it contains the enzymes of the pancreas (the immune organ) and Thymus, the training organ of the T-cells.

No wonder it is hailed as one of the most remarkable immune-system stimulating products. It is one of the best selling products in Germany and has been studied extensively and proven to be effective (to some degree) in many auto-immune diseases. These diseases run in bouts and are associated with a derailed immune system. We have discussed them previously in Chapter Three: rheumatoid arthritis, Crohn's disease, Bechterew's disease, colitis ulcerosa, Systemic Lupus Erythematodes (SLE), scleroderma, multiple sclerosis (M.S.) and others. What is the mechanism of these diseases? They are a consequence of the continuing existence of **immune complexes**. The development of these complexes is a reaction which occurs a thousand times daily. Whenever antigens, such as chemicals, viruses, yeast cells or bacteria, enter the body, they are being bound by antibodies. The reactionary product are immune complexes. Under normal conditions these immune complexes are neutralized and shortly after their development, eliminated again. They become dangerous when they are not eliminated, which is the case in auto-immune diseases. Immune complexes are deposited in the tissue, damaging the host's own cells. These deposits occur in the joints (causing rheumatoid arthritis); in the kidney (causing glomerulonephritis); in the intestines (resulting in Crohn's disease or colitis ulcerosa); or in the pancreas (leading to chronic recurring pancreatitis).

High doses of Polyzym O22 have been used in these conditions (10 tablets, 3 times daily), bringing favorable results and not causing the side-effects of cortisone preparations, the first-line drug in these diseases. In many patients long-lasting remissions were achieved for a duration of up to ten years.

In light of the effectiveness of Polyzym 022, Karl Ransberger, the manufacturer of these enzymes, has started a protocol for AIDS patients.The results are not yet known. But Polyzym O22 definitely results in a quick neutralizing of common cold viruses, shortening the course of flu in a dramatic way. Polyzym O22 seems to be on its way to playing an increasingly important role in the defense of our immune system.

3. EXERCISE, A MUST!

"I don't feel like it," I hear you say. "All I can do is cope with my work, but for the rest, I am a couch potato." If you suffer from CEBV or Candida, it might feel that way. The fatigue seems to overwhelm you, it is like a curtain closing on you. It does not help that we start the pattern of physical unfitness at a young age. While California with its year-round fair weather might be an exception, children elsewhere usually lack endurance and physical stamina. Obesity increases, as do cholesterol levels, and therefore heart disease looms over young adults. High blood pressure, the bane of elderly people, now hits our children. There are several reasons. First of all, we parents do not set the best example. We always seem to find a reason to **not** exercise: too much work, bad climate, too much drinking the previous evening and simply a lack of enthusiasm. Hardly a stimulus for our children. The schools don't seem to help either. In Europe, especially Germany, part of the day is dedicated to physical education. Here, most students get as little physical education as one hour a week. Smoking cigarettes is chic. The food in school cafeterias does not help much. Besides, children spend their lunch-money to buy candy, available at school, thereby decreasing the strength of their immune system. Thank God, with all the hype regarding cholesterol and heart disease, some efforts are being made to shape our children up. New exercise programs are being devised, there are some courses on "How to Choose Healthful Foods," and the "Say No to Drugs" program promotes also negative attitudes towards smoking.

If our children are shaping up, shouldn't we adults, follow their example? If you are healthy, don't take it for granted. An exercise routine should be part of your daily regimen. It does not have to be a preparation for the next Olympics. Too many people forget that they are out of shape and try to keep up with people who have exercised all their lives. Stress fractures, shin splints, tendonitis and other ailments are the immediate result, sidelining the victim for an undetermined time and convincing him that "exercise is not for him." Begin slowly. A twenty-minute workout, three times a week, jogging, walking, biking or swimming. Warm up before you start exercising, and even more important, do some stretching exercises **after** you are done with the exercise, in order to supply your activated muscles with blood. People are more motivated when they have "sparring" partners. I guess misery and pain love company. It is less boring, you are more motivated to do the exercise when you do it in pair, because you don't want to let your partner down. Once you see some results, you are on a "roll." Maybe you have been able to shed those pounds finally, or you feel fitter in your next tennis match; you require less sleep and you simply feel better emotionally. And the next blood test by your doctor might show decreased cholesterol levels.

What about exercise if you suffer from CEBV or Candida? I have already discussed this facet on page # 97. Even with these patients, exercise is a **must**. But do the exercise first thing in the morning, before shower and breakfast. Don't wait until later, because you will have less benefit from the exercise or simply you won't have any energy left. Why? Because during the night, especially when you take medication for those conditions, you will accumulate toxins, making your body heavy by the next morning. There is nothing better than having a sweat (except a good bowel movement) to release those toxins, and to make you pounds lighter. It is a wonderful start for the day. Often you might feel that you cannot put one foot in front of the other. Most people are pleasantly surprised, when they force themselves to exercise, that they feel so much better. Stationary bikes and rowing machines are popular gear in America's households, but walking is cheaper and beneficial to the heart and lungs as well. So if you think exercise is too strenuous, boring, unpleasant and only for "health nuts," think again -- because the enemies invading your immune system take plenty of exercise and strengthen **themselves** through mutations and innovative ways of penetrating into the core of your defense system. So stick to the golden rule: strike back through exercise!

4. INDOOR POLLUTION: HOW TO COMBAT IT?

Living in the Los Angeles area, I am painfully reminded every day of outdoor pollution. On hazy, smoggy days, when the beautiful mountains surrounding our valley disappear from sight, breathing becomes difficult, and eyes water, headaches and coughs become a constant reminder of the danger in our air. To avoid these toxic substances in the air, some people go to the beach, the mountains or the countryside, but the vast majority prefer to stay inside, in air-conditioned rooms. But is this such a wise alternative? Not if we can believe a report issued in 1984 by the Consumer Product Safety Commission. It states that indoor air pollution may be ten times **worse** than outdoor pollution.

Let's start with office buildings, a place where most of us spend most of our time. In thirty years, most new jobs will be white-collar jobs, and many of them will be involved in information processing. Links between workplace conditions and disease might be pretty obvious to the victim; however it is extremely easy for others to raise serious doubts about these connections. First of all, the effects might appear only years later, after chronic exposure. Secondly, the attitude among the manufacturers of chemicals is that they must be **proven** unsafe before being banned. In plain language, that means that you and I must first become sick, and then have the energy and money to prove that their products are the cause of our illness. Would it not be much fairer for the government to require those manufacturers to do extensive testing for toxicity before exposing us? No wonder immuno-suppressed diseases have become rampant.

What are the hazards we encounter in our offices? Poorly ventilated office buildings are at the top of the list. This is a direct result of the energy crisis in the mid-1970s, leading to a trend of energy-efficient designed buildings. These airtight buildings reduce heating and cooling costs. At the same time these offices recycle oxygen, but do not adequately filter it or mix it with fresh air. Because windows are scarce or do not open, workers breathe recycled air full of potential toxic vapors and cigarette smoke. What do you inhale? Asbestos from insulation, floor and ceiling tiles: the small dusty fibers can lodge in the lungs, irritate and inflame the lung mucosae at first, leading to crippling lung conditions with chronic exposure. It is strange, knowing that the dangers of asbestos are so well-documented, that we still are not looking for alternatives. Other pollutants are formaldehyde from glues and fabric, microorganisms in pipes and ventilation equipment, tobacco smoke and volatile compounds from cleaning and copying fluids and felt pens. With the omnipresence of copying machines in the modern workplace, workers are exposed to ozone, since the intense light of copying machines turns oxygen into ozone.

As if all this is not enough, computers have created a new challenge to our health. Modern technology has inundated us with these video display terminals (VDTs), and yet so little is known about their long-range effects on our health. However, short-term consequences are already visible: headaches, skin rashes, muscular pains and depression. This is not surprising when we know that these VDTs create an environment of positive ions, zapping the energy from their human operators.

Amid all these "enemies" in our offices, there is one additional danger above us: **lighting**. The damaging effects of poor building lighting on our health were extensively exposed by John Ott, author of "Health and Light." In spite of dramatic documentation regarding improvement in worker performance and reduction in absenteeism when full-spectrum lights are installed, very few offices have the ultraviolet wave lengths that are present in sunlight. It does not involve much expense to install these lights, but the gain to one's health is enormous. I know that it is going to take years of hard work by organized workers to convince government leaders of the "Sick Building Syndrome." Building owners have no incentive to improve working conditions, as long as their buildings are occupied. In the meantime, workers should open windows when this is possible. Bring green plants into your workplace, since they give off oxygen. Try to have a shield installed for your VDT and try to establish a cooperative relationship with your boss. After all, his health is also endangered. Installing full-spectrum lights is a must and rather inexpensive. In spite of all this, I am afraid that things will become worse before they get better. Maybe building owners have to be sued before they are willing to make mandatory changes. But we workers should not allow untested chemicals to steal our energy and health. Hard work, yes. Dangerous work, NO!

Just when we want to take refuge from our dangerous working conditions and restore our energy at home, bad news hits us here as well. While we have no problems "psyching" ourselves up for a fight against hazardous waste sites, few of us realize that the risk of getting cancer from exposure to chemicals in water and other solvents found in the home is far greater than the risk from exposure to those chemicals in waste sites. Here is a list of the enemies:

FORMALDEHYDE

RADON

ASBESTOS

COMBUSTION GASES,
ALLERGENS AND WATER POLLUTANTS

FORMALDEHYDE

This infamous product is present everywhere. It is used in the resins to make plywood and wood paneling; in the foam in urea formaldehyde insulation; in the adhesives used with carpeting and wallpaper; in paper products, permanent-press fabrics and hundreds of cosmetics. Reactions to exposure to formaldehyde are well-known: headaches, nausea, dizziness, insomnia and skin rashes. If you want to measure the formaldehyde level in your home, the 3-M Corporation, in White Bear Lake, Minn. (612-426-0691) sells a device (for around $50) that can measure the amount of formaldehyde in your rooms. In case the level exceeds the limit that the Federal Government has established, you can apply some simple strategies to reduce the amount of formaldehyde.

You can apply an epoxy sealer to plywood and fiberboards already in your house (epoxy is a non-toxic sealer). Another effective move is to buy more house plants, especially spider plants and philodendrons, since they absorb formaldehyde.

RADON

Decay products of Radon are one of the major causes of lung cancer. Radon diffuses out of rocks and soil and becomes a problem when it accumulates in an enclosed area such as a basement. Radon enters houses through cracks in foundations and basement floors. Again you can test your house for Radon contamination. You can get a measuring device from the "Radon Project, Department of Physics and Astronomy, University of Pittsburgh, PA. 15260. Sealing cracks will reduce to some extent the Radon levels, but sometimes a special ventilation system has to be installed.

ASBESTOS

This "wonder product" used in almost all buildings between 1920 and 1970 is also highly carcinogenic if fibers are released into the air. Lung cancer and an irreversible lung disease, asbestosis, are consequences. One finds asbestos used in insulation of walls, to strengthen vinyl floors and to fireproof walls. The Federal Government has prohibited its use since the '70s, but many older houses have these sources of asbestos which need to be removed by professsionals.

COMBUSTION GASES and ALLERGENS

The best thing you can do is to get rid of your gas stove and replace it with an electric one. Build up of CO2 or Carbon Dioxide causes headaches, dizziness, nausea and impaired memory. If you have a gas stove, try to replace it with one without a pilot light or one that functions through spark ignition. The flames have to burn blue instead of orange. More than once we have read about tragedies where CO2 killed families who were heating their houses with their gas ovens: they literally asphyxated themselves.

Another major source of asphyxation is inhalation of dust

particles. Dust contains viruses, bacteria and mites, ready to attack any weakness in your immune system. You have several solutions: negative ionizers and electrostatic precipators are helpful; but no air purifier is as important as cleaning your house. People with allergies should also stay away from dogs and cats, or at least keep them out of the bedroom. And wash your bedding, pillows and drapes with a 1% tannic acid solution. They will remain hypoallergenic even after repeated washings with detergents.

WATER POLLUTANTS

The purchase of a water purifier will be an investment in your future health. According to the EPA, two percent of the country's community water supply poses a significant risk to human health. If you have questions about the safety of your water, call the EPA's toll-free number (800) 426-4791. One of the problems is to choose the right water purifier for your house. The National Sanitation Foundation, 3475 Plymouth Road, Ann Harbor, Mich. 48106, has a list of the most effective ones.

It is clear from the above that we have a hard and sometimes expensive battle in front of us. As more and more people with immuno-suppressed diseases become reactive and sensitive to the environment, the need for "non-toxic" houses will increase. Some architects and contractors are already specializing in this: they use low-toxic or non-toxic materials for particle boards, wallpaper glue and paint, and insulation made of cork. The price is about twenty percent higher than for conventional houses, but for the millions of people already suffering from allergies, it is worth it. Considering the cancers and other irreversible conditions toxic house materials causes, it seems a small investment in your health.

5. ACUPUNCTURE AND HOMEOPATHY: THE RETURN TO ANCIENT MEDICINES TO HELP SOLVE OUR MODERN PROBLEMS.

I have already discussed extensively the value of acupuncture in boosting the immune system (See Chapter One, Page # 32). It is clear that with people increasingly reacting to preservatives in medications, a pure and natural art such as acupuncture can only gain in value for the immuno-suppressed patient. With the increase of T-Helper cells, the increased phagocytic activity and the improvement in endocrine and hormone function, acupuncture definitely has a place in the treatment program of the immuno deficient patient.

The history of homeopathic treatment is a similar one. It does not have as long a lifespan as acupuncture, but considerably longer than conventional Western medicine. Dr. Samuel Hahneman was one of Napoleon Bonaparte's doctors. On his route to conquer most of Europe, Napoleon used the innovative skills of Dr. Hahneman to keep his troops free of typhoid fever. Hahneman created a totally new concept of medicine, which he called "Homeopathy," derived from the Greek words, "homeos," which means "similar," and, "pathos" or "disease." Hahneman's basic law was, "Let's cure a disease with the disease itself, or like cures like." His theory had and still has an enormous following in Europe. In France, Belgium and Holland, you can find thousands of M.D.'s trained in homeopathy. In England, the Royal Mother's physician is a homeopath. Even in the USA, homeopathy was practiced by a large number of physicians until it was removed from the medical scene by the powerful pharmaceutical companies and the AMA.

There are major differences between homeopathy and conventional medicine. For one, homeopathy **never** has side-efffects; conventional medicine **always** has. Homeopathy is cheap, conventional medicine is expensive. Homeopathy treats the patient in a way that supports the immune system, whereas conventional medicine often blocks the natural defense mechanisms (cortisone being a perfect example). Homeopathy treats the cause; conventional medications often are purely symptomatic (think of anti-fever and anti-rheumatic medications). In other words, the symptom in homeopathy is considered a defensive reaction, one that tries to overcome the invader; the homeopathic programs the body to heal **itself**, quite the contrary to conventional medicine where the doctor tries to counter what is happening, often hampering the body's natural defense system. The diagnosis in homeopathy largely depends on a painstaking inquiry, often as long as two hours, where physical **and** mental symptoms are taken into consideration. In conventional medicine, we are relying mostly on complicated and sophisticated lab tests, a lot of them non-specific and not sensitive enough, prompting incorrect diagnosis and treatment. The Candida epidemic is a consequence of this. Modern medicine all too often views the mind and body as two separately functioning entities, to be treated by different doctors. Homeopathic doctors as well as acupuncturists are holistic doctors, observing and respecting the body-mind unit. Therefore, the object of homeopathic treatment is a permanent resolution of the condition.

Inevitably, with the rising incidence of the immuno-suppressed diseases, incapable of being cured by conventional medicine, homeopathic treatment is on the increase. I predict that by the year 2000, 80% of the conventional pharmacologic therapeutics will be replaced by homeopathy.

6. PRACTICAL TREATMENT PLAN FOR THE IMMUNO-SUPPRESSED PATIENT

1. Step one: DIAGNOSTIC TESTS

. CBC & differential, thyroid panel and chemscreen

. Immune panel (as outlined on page # 64)

. CEIA test

. 3 day stool culture test for parasites

. EBV panel (IgG, NA, VCA, and IgM)

. CMV and other Herpes Simplex IgG levels

. HIV test

. Take the basal temperature under the armpit, to exclude low thyroid function (first thing in the morning, temperature has to be between 97.8 and 98.2).

2. Step 2: TREAT THE UNDERLYING CONDITION FIRST

The above tests will give enough information to determine the direction of treatment. All underlying conditions should be corrected if possible, **first**, before even attempting to boost the immune system.

3. Step 3: INTRODUCE A CORRECT DIET

All immuno-suppressed patients should start the diet as outlined in this chapter. An immune system cannot get boosted without a healthy diet.

4. Step 4: BOOST THE IMMUNE SYSTEM WITH SUPPLEMENTS, HOMEOPATHY AND ACUPUNCTURE.

Usually after treating the underlying factors for about six weeks, one should start boosting the immune system with the supplements outlined earlier.

7

OPEN LETTER TO THE "FAMILY" OF THE ENVIRONMENTAL, IMMUNO-SUPPRESSED PATIENT

INTRODUCTION

I have addressed this message to the "family" of immuno-suppressed patients, and I mean the extended family: spouses, gentlemen-friends, lady-friends, casual friends and yes, the occasional person these patients might meet at parties or on dining occasions. While this chapter might be helpful for the "family," I hope it also provides a tool for the patient. Candida and CEBV patients have to defend themselves continously against disbelief, rejection and insults: laziness, self-centeredness and immaturity are charges leveled at them on every occasion.

While I hope that the previous chapters have shown amply to what degree these victims suffer, I want to demonstrate the flip side of the coin: the "family" that is frightened, unable to answer the cry for help, that feels manipulated and "unloved" by the sufferer. While knowledge of the disease is a big step forward in securing the support of friends, it takes a lot more to really help: it takes unconditional love. And this was the lesson I learned.

MY OWN "REAL" UNDERSTANDING

In my practice I was giving support and treatment to thousands of immuno-suppressed patients. I thought I was doing a good job. I thought I, more than anybody else, understood these patients. I felt empathy for them, I could cry with them, I could feel the desperation in their soul. I could hear the cry for help. I felt like a rock upon which these patients could stand. Sometimes, I became enraged by the injustice done to these patients by their own families, by the indifference of parents who, rather than being there for their child, would go into hiding and deny the problem. The subject of the child's disease was taboo. Obvious signs of distress were dismissed with well-meant remarks such as, "If you would just grow up," "If you would only mature and take a job like everybody else." I thought to myself: "How can they be so heartless, where is the parental love these children deserve?" It was rather judgmental on my part. In my practice, I was with these sufferers for at least eight hours a day, being doctor, friend, therapist or just a substitute for the "family member" they were looking for.

I failed to see one thing: I went home after work into an entirely different atmosphere and I lived a completely different life. I could go to the theatre, play tennis, go dancing, have dinner with friends... it was all possible. It took my personal involvement in their lives to come to a full understanding of the suffering of both the patients and their families. It was not until I met a friend, S., that I fully understood the suffering of the patient as well as that of his family. Here I was, confronted for the first time, with the reality of Candida and environmental hypersensitivity. I realized that the name of the problem was **ENERGY.**

Energy is the one word that dominates the lives of immuno-suppressed patients. These victims do not have energy, or even more devastating, they never know when they will have energy. They feel rotten today, but hope for a good day tomorrow, so that they can put some order into their lives. Yet when tomorrow comes, there is again no energy. The reasons are various: the patient may react to a previous treatment; she can be premenstrual; there is suddenly a reaction to a new food; or he becomes ill from automobile exhaust while driving. In fact, the causes are unlimited, and sometimes hard to pin down. Emotional traumas, often present, don't help neither. So instead of a whole day, the patient can count on only one-third of the day, the other two-thirds being needed for rest, to sit still, waiting for the small rally in mental and physical strength. Sometimes the latter does not come for a whole week, and the daily chores pile up, increasing the anxiety in the patient, especially when the spouse comes home and says: "You had the whole day, what did you do?"

This is the difficult part for the family to understand: the patient did not have the whole day; she might have had two hours of that day. It is very hard for a healthy person to understand this, and it is easy to become irritated with the "lazy" behavior of the victim. But there is no way the patient can push herself beyond a certain point: she will pay tenfold for it the next day. So if there are two hours of energy left in a day, the patient is forced to use them for everybody and everything else -- the long-waiting chores, the friend that absolutely had to see her, the spouse that wanted to see that movie. But no time was left for her own needs. There are only two things dominating her life: reacting to the disease or the treatments, and spending her remaining energy on everything else but herself. Not a very easy way to live and not a life-style that is conducive to healing. The patient feels worthless and the family feels left out of her world. The disease rules the family.

HOW DID I REACT?

I am ashamed to say that I did not do much better than the average person would have done. I could not understand why my friend did not want to be with me as much as I wanted to be with her. Did she not love me as much as I loved her? Why didn't she want me to come to visit when she wasn't feeling well? I tried to persuade her, pleaded with her, in short I pressured her. Sometimes I persuaded her to let me come anyway, in spite of her not feeling well. I finally wore her down by saying,"I'll be there just for you, you don't have to be 'up' for me." However, when I was with her, I encountered for the first time the total lack of affection that must be present in a crisis with these patients. She had such a hard time just dealing with herself, that there was no room for me or anything else.

Did I understand that I was not the target of this attitude? I had difficulty with it. I could sometimes talk to her without getting an answer. It irritated me. Didn't I go out of my way to help her? I deserved better, I thought. I did not understand that the need for her to rely on me was stressful in itself. Family members take note: those patients do not like the position of dependency that they are put in, they hate it! And although you might think, "I am doing all I can, and I don't deserve this treatment," the patients are the ones who suffer the most. They gladly would trade places with you. After all, they don't have any choice; you, on the other hand, have plenty of choices. You can go out with a friend, have dinner in a restaurant or engage in your favorite sport. Your family-victim will just have to wait for some good moments.

HOW DID I GET THE HELP "I" NEEDED?

The first help I received was from myself. I wanted to be with S., and I wanted to help her. However, reading some pertinent books she gave me, I began to understand that my "love" was very limited. Sure, I loved her as long as she behaved the way I wanted her to. The moment I had some expectations and she did not read my mind or could "not perform," I was disappointed. My own ego and pain were in the way. In fact, it was my ego that dictated my defensive behavior. Whatever subject came up, I would read between the lines, feel attacked and unloved, and feel justified in retaliating.

I should have known better: the words "attack" and "battle" and even more "ego," leave no place for love. In fact, the goal of the ego is to defeat love. This relationship took quite an adjustment, lots of pain and sadness. But it was worth it, no matter what the outcome would be. I knew I was only at the beginning of a road I had never traveled before: the road to unconditional love and inner peace. I knew it was going to be a hard journey, a long process. It taught me several valuable lessons that all of us can use to help an immuno-suppressed patient. I do not presume to force them upon any of my readers; I simply state that I tried to focus on them, repeating them to myself every day. I called them my nine daily check points.

THE NINE DAILY CHECK POINTS

1. Practice unconditional love

This is really the only rule, the most complete one and maybe the most difficult one to follow. Ninety five percent of all existing relationships are controlling, based on fears and conditions. "I love you, but...," or "I love you as long as you behave the way I want you to behave." Let there be no ifs, ands or buts! Unconditional love, found in any loving relationship, is the purest form of love. You love your partner or friend, with all the weaknesses and handicaps that they have, you accept them for what they are. Of course, this does not mean you should take emotional or physical abuse. The latter are not precisely signs of love, but rather of a disturbed personality. You can use your love to steer your partner in the right direction, and to lend your full support if he or she is willing to change.

2. Love and forgive yourself

If you want to give love to the patient in your family, you had better start loving yourself. You might think you have contributed to the disease of your spouse, and sometimes you may have. You might feel guilty for not being able to help your spouse and find yourself trying to escape the situation. Say goodbye to guilt, forgive yourself and love yourself. You cannot possibly give love if you feel that you deserve no love. Time and time again, you may fall into the trap of defensiveness, telling yourself that you don't deserve a spouse who is such a burden.

3. Forget the negative check-list

I have caught myself many times concentrating on some small negative characteristics of my friend. As a result, small remarks became monstrous, snowballing until they exploded, leaving us both in a daze. It is so easy to focus on those negative facts, because they allow us to avoid the work needed to improve the relationship. The check-list of faults inevitably becomes bigger and bigger until it takes on monstrous proportions, overshadowing any potential joy. Focus instead on the positive points of your partner. Sometimes even in their extreme illness, people can contribute to society if they are allowed to do so and find a support group.

4. Do some fun things with friends

Family members do occasionally catch the immuno-suppressed disease from the patient. I don't mean simply physically, but also emotionally. Most of the time there is no energy to go to restaurants, enjoy sports or go to parties. Environmental sensitivities exclude an evening at the theater, because your hypersensitive spouse might have a seat next to somebody wearing a heavy perfume. You feel like a prisoner. It takes understanding of the patient this time to allow the spouse to have some fun time with friends. As long as the action involved does not harm the relationship and the commitment to the partner is honored, it should take away some pressure from the situation, leaving room to breathe for both people involved. Having his or her batteries recharged, a spouse can dedicate fresh energy to the patient and actually have more empathy and compassion.

5. Get a therapist on your team

For everyone involved in the family of a hypersensitive patient, a counselor is not only welcome help but a must. Especially for the patient -- for the chance to unload the frustration of not being able to contribute more to society or family, for the guilt for being such a "pest," and for the mood swings fluctuating sometimes to suicidal proportions. Also the rest of the family needs to "unload" their frustration, because there is no way that the sick person, who requires all his energy for survival, will be able to carry them, too. The therapist, knowing both parties, can give suggestions. Being non-judgmental and not siding with either one of the parties, he or she will be an intermediary help in to establish cohesiveness, which is necessary for the healing of each individual involved.

6. Be honest with yourself

The first thing I had to do in coping with this problem was take an honest look at myself. Why did I react the way I did? I caught myself reacting in an insensitive way, as though I did not understand the situation and could not summon any empathy. I could not be the support my friend needed until I first resolved my own issues. This is the reason why a therapist is absolute necessary; don't think you are smart enough to resolve your own painful issues. Understanding yourself will lead to better acceptance of your partner, bring you closer, and strengthen you in handling any future problem.

7. Give the sick person space

As already mentioned, energy is the name of the game. If the patient needs to withdraw and be by herself, let her. Don't push her, because then she will have to spend precious energy trying to explain why she cannot accommodate you. No matter what, the result for you will be the same, she will not be able to go along with your desires. For the victim, the outcome will not be the same: exhausted because of the efforts to explain, she will require extra time to recuperate -- precious time she could have spent with you or on some worthy goal. This necessity for space will vary from person to person, but also from time to time within the same person. During the premenstrual period, for instance, the need for withdrawal will be greater.

8. Be a team player

This is not in the least a minor rule. You can show understanding by sharing a special diet with the patient. You might be surprised how tasteful it is, how much more energy it will give you, and simply, how pleasant it can be to be innovative. Sharing in this way removes the burden of making two separate dinners. Besides, if the patient has cravings, it is no fun for her to see the other person gubbling down forbidden goodies. Actually, a very interesting phenomenon can occur. Usually my patients are well-motivated to follow the diet, but some of them receive "static" from their partners for doing so. What happens is that the other person feels guilty about his own lousy diet; it makes him think about it. So if you are someone's partner don't sabotage the diet by buying all the wrong foods. Instead, start looking at the healthful food around you and try to develop a taste for that.

Being a team player is not restricted to food intake. Exercise together, stop smoking and drinking, and stay away from drugs.

Help the patient organize and execute some of those daily routines; it feels very good to the patient when the daily check-list gets shorter instead of longer.

Even more important in helping the recovery of your spouse is getting tested yourself for Candida or CEBV. Patients can work very hard to overcome these chronic conditions, and they relapse because they get reinfected by their spouses. I have seen it happen many times. You can imagine the frustration and even rage of patients, being sabotaged in their hard, long road to personal healing. So be the team player you promised to be when you entered your relationship.

9. Try to communicate better

Sometimes the patient already feels so guilty that s/he does not want to express certain wishes. The other partner, feeling so many times "rejected," stops asking and assumes that the partner will guess his or her desires. Anger is the next step after not being understood. In fact, what happens often is that verbal communication becomes very difficult, because the other party always thinks that there is an "attack," so self-defense is in order.

Conversations like that lead only to the destruction of any good feeling in the relationship. So if you have come to the point where verbal communication becomes impossible, write each other a letter. And write the whole truth, everything that you would like to express: your anger, frustration, fear, but also your wishes, desires, hopes and love. In fact, make sure you start with the negative feelings, and finish with the positive ones. Be sure the harsh feelings don't outweigh the positive ones.

I hope this "Open Letter" can bring some understanding to both parties. Let's face it. If your relationship survives an immuno-suppressed disease, it will survive almost anything!

How was the outcome in my relationship? I was not able to hold on. In fact, I believe that it is extremely hard to build up a relationship since the opportunities to do so are non-existant. How can you get to know each other when you can't do things together? Relationships are built upon common interests, shared pleasures and experiences. It is different when you have already a relationship through marriage before the disease hits. You have known your partner before, there is already a bond. Sadly enough, a lot of marriages strand on the cliff of these diseases. Therefore, this open letter is especially aimed at people in an existing relationship. If the immuno-suppressed patient does not have a relationship, I advise him not to enter one. You will save both parties alot of sadness. Let that patient focus on her recovery, she will need all the energy she has left.

8

ANCIENT MEDICINES COMBINED: THE POSSIBLE WAY OUT!

It is obvious from the previous chapters that modern medicine has its back to the wall as far as immuno-suppressed conditions are concerned. In spite of millions of dollars of research, we are losing ground to viruses, bacterias and yeast cells: these invaders have joined forces to relentlessly attack the bodies of their victims. When you think you conquered one condition, another related one appears and demands immediate attention from your already weakened immune system. It is already difficult to find a person between the age of 20 and 45 who does not suffer from either one of the Herpes Simplex family viruses, parasites or yeast cells. Unless we drastically change our environment and life style, I predict that in a few years it will be impossible to find a person free of any of these immuno-suppressed diseases. Since many of these conditions can be easily transferred, there seems to be no mechanism available to stop this snowball effect. If we ever are going to make a stand, we have to do it **now!**

We have already discussed the environmental and life style changes that are imperative to deal with the greatest threat of this century. Only after such changes, will new medications be of significant help in putting down these hordes of invaders. I have always been convinced that whatever disease might be lurking around the corner, the remedy can be found in nature. Nature has provided us with magnificent tools, yet most of them remain undiscovered. In Europe, ancient arts of medicine such as acupuncture, herbology and homeopathy, have been incorporated in our therapeutic modalities with great success. Even more exciting, different modalities have been combined: injections of vitamins or herbs in carefully selected acupuncture points were performed in Holland, France and Germany for years with often stunning results. It is this approach that will bring hope to all of you sufferers, who had to first overcome years of frustration because of disbelief, and finally, when the condition was recognized and validated, had to struggle to find an efficient therapy.

WHAT IS SO EXCITING ABOUT THIS NEW APPROACH?

One of the pitfalls of modern interventionary medicine, is that side-effects are always present. This makes it hard often for patients who are in the most urgent need to get efficient therapy. The practice of medicine becomes a negotiating process: will we try to eradicate one condition at the price of creating another one in the future? Often such a choice is made because doctors and patients want immediate results, and are willing to worry about longterm side-effects later. Up until now, we always got away with it -- although with sometimes sad consequences. Millions of people are addicted to sleeping pills and pain killers, or suffer the devastating consequences of chronic cortisone therapies. Aside from these health consequences, medications are expensive, draining the coffers of the family, producing resentment, sadness and despair. Look at AZT, hailed as the only helpful medication in AIDS (inspite of its side-effects): the marketing pharmaceutical company makes it available at a prohibitive cost.

It is clear that for chronic, debilitating conditions such as CEBV or Candida, we need inexpensive, effective and safe medications. Let's not put our victims into two camps: one that can afford treatment, the other that can't.

This is where homeopathy enters: we have already discussed (Chapter 6), how safe, inexpensive and effective this treatment is. What is homeopathy? It is not a question of **delusions** but **dilutions!** In short terms, homeopathy is the use of minute doses of drugs that bring on symptoms similar to the disease to stimulate a cure. For example, it is possible to dilute an aqueous solution of an antibody indefinitely without the solution losing its biological activity. Strangely enough, at some dilutions the activity falls off; on further dilution, it is restored. Samual Hahnemann, a German physician of the late 1700s, built the homeopathic treatment around the "law of similars", which held that the power of a drug to cure a disease is related to its ability to produce symptoms of the disease itself. However, Hahnemann also believed that the body's healing mechanisms could be triggered by a very small doses of a drug, or combinations of drugs. And that is precisely what is used in homeopathic modern treatments: herbal products, diluted in homeopathic doses, leaving behind spiritlike substances that set in motion the body's "vital force" or QI.

Recently, the British journal **Nature** published a study that supports the homeopathic theory. In the report, a French allergist, Jacques Benveniste of the University of Paris-Sud, found that white blood cells, basophils, react to an antibody solution after the equivalent of 120 tenfold dilutions. Up to 60% of the basophil membranes were disrupted by these weak solutions. It was as if these homeopathic solutions remembered their earlier larger concentrations. The publishers of **Nature** were so startled by these results that they waited two years before publishing them. How did the medical world react? As usual, they asked for more proof, more studies. However, the homeopathic researchers are confident enough that they have announced that they will do controlled studies, and the second run of the experiment will appear in a later edition of **Nature.** The second team, visiting Dr. J. Benvenistes lab came to a total different conclusion. They found that the claims made by this doctor, were "based on experiments which were ill-controlled." One has to wonder what they based their opinion on. The pressure from the medical community? Incompetence? I find it strange that the visiting team of Nature, consituted of a professional magician(!), a journalist with a background in theoretical physics and another person familiar with the misconduct in scientific literature. In my opinion, hardly a group to judge highly experienced researchers who founded their findings on five years of hard work. It is always the same: how can you discuss certain methods with people who know nothing about the science itself? It is interesting to note that the art of Homeopathy was tested in a double-blind method by medical doctors of the Glasgow University. Their results appeared in the most respected medical magazine in Europe,"The Lancet, (October 18, '86)." The overal conclusion was that "patients taking a homeopathic preparation showed a greater improvement in symptoms than those taking a placebo." We have to remember that throughout history, a great deal of progress in science has come from unorthodox ideas. It is much better to err on the side of publishing potential new ideas than of suppressing potentially worthwhile life saving remedies.

Acupuncture and its laws have been discussed in Chapter One. Imagine the combination of homeopathy and acupuncture. And that's the idea: herbal products diluted in homeopathic dosage, and injected in acupuncture points. The result is phenomenal. It is totally safe: the dilution in homeopathic strength makes it available to any age group and to the most sensitive patient, because homeopathic dilutions are so small that they cannot be measured by normal laboratory standards. Yet, in this lies their strength. By injecting these solutions into carefully selected acupuncture points, we are able to telegraph this information (because that's what it is), to the organ that is weak.

WHAT ARE THE RESULTS?

It often happens that the patient feels an IMMEDIATE effect on the treatment table. A sense of well-being, a clearing up of the brain fog, a surge of energy and a feeling of being centered for the first time in a long while. Frequently, the next day a Herxheimer or die-off reaction is experienced. Some headaches, flu-like symptoms and fatigue, relieved by a good bowel movement. The die-off reaction might last for two to ten days, after which the patient feels a higher level of energy and clear headedness.

There are numerous advantages to this method. Besides the low cost and lack of side-effects, this kind of treatment takes only a couple of months, where previous treatments for Candida for example, with nystatin, capricin or tanalbit, take at least from six months to two years. Not a very encouraging thought when you have to change your diet for that long. Don't misunderstand me. I want my patients to change their diet permanently. Nobody with a clear head on his shoulders wants to stuff sugar, preservatives and coloring substances in his body. But it is a relief to most patients that they can start adding wheat, rye, yoghurt and additional fruits to their diet already after about six weeks.

The speed with which we are achieving results is also very encouraging. Each treatment brings major changes when the patient follows the well-outlined program. After the initial die-off period, every week groups of previous symptoms decrease in intensity or disappear. It is very encouraging when the digestion starts working properly, when there are days that the energy level is up or when one can think clearly for the first time. I have had patients who could not follow psychotherapy because they were unable to focus or come in contact with their feelings. After a couple of treatments, they felt as though a curtain were lifted, a whole new world opened for them. Many patients become very emotional during the therapy, because coming into touch with hidden anger, frustration and sadness can be very painful. But at last, they can work on those issues, because they are able to feel them.

There is one danger that I see: patients are so encouraged by the results that they let up too early. They feel so energetic, free from dizzy attacks and bloating, that they think they can go overboard with certain foods too early in the program. The awakening is rude. Immediate headaches, bloating, constipation and brain fog are the result. Fortunately, they can rebound immediately if they get back on track again. We must not forget, that during this cleansing period, we are extremely sensitive to any bad foodstuff we want to bring into our systems. In fact, we will react with more severe symptoms to the same foods than during the period when we were really sick. It is simply, our body telling us: "don't add this junk to me while you are in the process of cleansing me."

How long does the treatment last? The major part of the treatment is complete in about 5 treatments with a 7 day interval between each injection. Afterwards, there will be a follow-up visit after 3 weeks. More frequent injections might be required depending on the individual case, because each case of Candida and CEBV is different. The make-up of these autoimmune deficiency conditions is so complex that no one patient is alike. Therefore, follow-up by a well-trained physician is absolutely necessary in order to make changes in the course of the treatment. It is obvious that the patient will have to adhere to a healthy lifestyle in order to boost the immune system, once the titers of EBV and Candida begin to drop.

WHAT ARE THE HERBS WE CAN USE IN DILUTED DOSES?

Let's start with the fight against Candida. In principal we can use any fungus killer present in nature. Well-proven fungus killers are Pau D'Arco (discussed page # 134), Hydrogen Peroxide (page # 133), Dioxichlor (page # 133) and Ausralian TEA TREE OIL or Melaleuca Alternifolia. The last one needs some further clari-fication.

Virtually unknown in the United States, Tea Tree oil has a long history. It was the observation of Aboriginals that led to an investigation of these trees, and to the discovery of the unique properties of the essential oil in Melaleuca alternifolia. The oil is a natural essential one, which is a safe, powerful, broad spectrum antiseptic and fungicide. It has a pleasant odor and is non-toxic, and non-irritating to normal tissue. The oil is distilled from the leaves of Melaleuca alternifolia, a tree species which grows in the remote and rugged bush swampland of the north coast of New South Wales. It gained its name from Joseph Banks, a botanist who joined Captain Cook in his first visit of discovery to Australia. He learned from the Aboriginal people that a delicious tea could be brewed from the leaves of certain trees, to which they attributed powerful medicinal and tonic effects.

The use of this anti-fungal has been known for quite some time in Europe. A study done by Dr. Paul Belaiche, head of the Phytotherapy Department at the college of Medicine of Bobigny (Paris) showed that the Tea Tree oil was active against Trichomonas vaginalis and Moniliasis. This was confirmed by another study done by Eduardo Pena, M.D., F.A.C.O.G. in 1961, published in the journal of Obstetrics and Gynecology, here in the United States.

Melaleuca has a powerful anti-mycotic action which is very well tolerated by the vaginal mucous membranes in case it is applied vaginally. It allows therefore a lengthy course of treatment which leads to the eradication of Candida. One can state that Melaleuca has entered the team of the essential oils and emerges as an anti-mycotic weapon of the first order in Natural Medicine.

The herbs used for CEBV and other Herpes Simplex viruses are similar in nature. Dioxychlor and Hydrogen Peroxide can both be used as single agents or combined to fight these viruses. Other herbs with known anti-viral properties are Rheum. Palmatum, Forsythia suspensa and Isatis tintoria. Knowing that antiviral therapy is a formidable challenge for modern medicine which has hardly produced a treatment against viruses period, the discovery of the anti-viral properties of these products has provided mankind with new hope in its fight against an omnipresent enemy.

With this particularly treatments I have helped thousands of patients successfully where any other treatment failed. In light of the enormous proportions that these conditions take, it comes as a light in the darkness. My hope is that it will become available throughout the United States, a standard tool in any medical practice.

CONCLUSION

Some people still may think that immuno-suppressed diseases are diseases of the future. It must be clear by now to the readers of this book that they are already reality for millions of people, and because of the stubborn nonacceptance of this reality by the medical profession, they will become the next nightmare in countless of individuals' lives.

But there is one positive aspect of this situation: it may force a change of attitude in medical profession. Suddenly there is no "magic bullet" available to wipe out these strange diseases. The variety of symptoms puzzles the medical community. "It is a fad disease." "A good psychiatrist is what you need. " These" quickie" solutions will not be good enough advice for the multitudes of sufferers stricken at the peak of their active lives. In fact, I predict that these victims will no longer tolerate such insults, but instead will seek the help of true healers, finding the support they need and deserve.

It is also clear that the task of facing these immuno-suppressed diseases is a formidable challenge for the patients. I think that their biggest mistake is that they make the disease the "absolute ruler" in their lives, to whom everything else must give way. Acting this way causes patients to lose control over their lives, so that they cannot commit themselves to the true goal of recovery. Of course, it is hard after years of suffering to think positively about yourself, or to believe that somebody still cares about you. In fact, it is hard even to love yourself.

This lack of self-esteem sets up a dangerous pattern of guilt. First, the patient feels guilty because s/he cannot participate in a constructive way in family life. More money is spent on special diets, doctors' visits and medications, funds that could have been used for more "meaningful" purposes. On the other hand, non-compliance with the diet and exercise program evokes a feeling of guilt, putting the patient in a "double-bind" no-win situation. Patients need to set realistic, positive goals, accepting the challenges facing them. You either face each obstacle with despair, depression and anger, or you see it as one more enemy to conquer. Look for the humor in the situation, share your feelings with family members and have hope, love and faith.

Another obstacle between the patient and his recovery is the way we habitually view medicine and its therapeutic modalities. We are used to getting immediate responses to a treatment: we take a pain pill, and the discomfort disappears rapidly. We can't sleep, but we are given a sleeping pill that allows us to get the necessary rest. We always know the approximate length of time before our disease runs its course. Healing a fracture will take from 4-6 weeks, a flu will last a week, and so on. This is perhaps the most frustrating aspect of the immuno-suppressed diseases. "How long is this going to last," and "When will I be feeling better or cured" are the most frequently asked questions. It is impossible to give an answer. Too much depends on the willingness of the patient to change his or her life style, something that is not always required in Western medicine, or at least not enough stressed by the medical community. Most of the time there are several immuno-suppressed conditions battling the patients' immune system. Moreover, patients generally tend to underestimate these conditions. That makes them impatient and irritable, emotions not very conducive to boost the immune system! We have to learn to look at each step we improved and not trying to jump to the end point, a goal we cannot see.

It is obvious to me that things will get worse before they get better. It is also clear that we have faulty priorities. How else can you explain the fact that we expend technical and financial resources to create preservatives, pesticides, bombs and nuclear plants, when millions of people die each year from malnutrition? This environmental pollution is poison to our spirits and hearts as well as our bodies, and we simply must not accept pollution as the normal.

As outlined in previous chapters, immuno-suppressed disseases have no single known cause, so that the dream of a single cure for them is just that, a dream. Western medicine has an obsession with "objectivity." Alas, our "objectivity" with its demand for "double-blind controls" leads to many failures.We have only to recall coronary by-pass operations, which became extremely popular in the Seventies, performed as the procedure to extend life, and provide patients with many extra rewarding years. However, a study done by the AMA itself concluded that after 10 years there was no significant difference in survival time between patients who had been operated on and patients who had not. Does this stop those operations? Absolutely not! They continue at almost the same "epidemic" rate.

We have become increasingly technical, forgetting that medicine remains an art, where the true healer has to master his technique in the same way as a great artist does. We must not forget that there is an important interaction between healer and patient. It will become ever more evident in the future that emotions are one of the most important factors at triggering diseases that affect our lives.

Illness of a part of the body does affect the whole. If a doctor fails to treat this unity, s/he treats the patient improperly and incompletely. You cannot subdivide human beings into small parcels and believe that all those magnificent technical advances will structure a perfect creature. We have to encourage love more. Love dissolves anger, it heals because it defuses a dangerous situation.

True healing is giving, without restraints of peer pressure and personal desire such as making quick money. The true healer of the future will fuse in his practice ancient methods (acupuncture, homeopathy) with new technical advantages, but always with one goal in mind: he will give himself to the patient with his whole heart and all his compassion. The only loyalty we should have is toward one another, with the ultimate goal: serving each other and life!

ORDERFORM

Please send ( ) copy (ies) of the book

"CANDIDA"
The symptoms, the causes, the cure

Unit price: $10.00
Postage: $2.50
CA residents add 7% sales tax

Ship to:

Name: ______________________________

Street: ______________________________

City: ________________ State: ________ Zip: ________

Total purchase amount: $

❑ Check enclosed

Charge my ❑ Visa ❑ Master card

Card # ______________________________

Expiration date ____________ phone (—) ____________

Signature ______________________________

MAIL TO:

Dr. Luc De Schepper, 2901 Wilshire Boulevard, Suite 435 Santa Monica, CA 90403

ORDERFORM

Please send ( ) copy (ies) of the book

"PEAK IMMUNITY"

Unit price: $15.00
Postage: $2.50

CA residents add 7% sales tax

Ship to:

Name: ____________________

Street: ____________________

City: ____________ State: ______ Zip: ______

Total purchase amount: $

❑ Check enclosed

Charge my ❑ Visa ❑ Master card

Card # ____________________

Expiration date ________ phone (—) ________

Signature ____________________

MAIL TO:

Dr. Luc De Schepper,
2901 Wilshire Boulevard, Suite 435
Santa Monica, CA 90403